The A to Z of Bone & Joint Failure

Introduction

When *the A to Z of Bones, Joints & Ligaments* was first written, I received requests to add an additional section dealing exclusively with the BACK. Hence, *the A to Z of the Bones, Joints, Ligaments & the Back* was written. was written. This was well received, and generated a interest in the common features & failings of bones & joints. Normal bone re-models itself constantly and this feature is the cause of osteoporosis and other bone/joint pathologies, when it goes awry. This is the first time the A to Z format has been applied to a purely pathological topic. The title was in part suggested by Prof John Eisman who is very concerned with the devastating problem of Osteoporosis. After discussions with him, and also with Prof Barry Wren, and feedback - the idea of a book on the failure of aspects of the skeletal system was born, hence this small volume. It is the first in a series of *the A to Z of ..... failure*. The next one planned is a discussion on the failings of the cardiovascular system, *The A to Z of Cardiovascular failure*.

Acknowledgement

Thank you Aspenpharmacare Australia for your support and assistance in this valuable project, particularly Greg Lan, and Rob Koster, and everyone who provided feedback. It is always greatly appreciated.

Dedication

I am lucky to have a small group around me who are supportive and loyal. Thank you. You know who you are!!! and of course to my A to Z darlings, who may be far away but are always on my mind. You know, I love you.

How to use this book

A basic anatomical knowledge of the Bones Joints & their associated structures is assumed in this book, and summarized in *the A to Z of Bones Joints, Ligaments & the Back*. There are 2 main sections in this book: a consideration of the normal tissues and the latter green section - a consideration of their pathological processes. The Appendix summarizes the major bone diseases as a table.

The Common Terms section also includes a number of pathological terms and diagrams.

This book is cross-referenced with all the other A to Zs.

The A to Zs may be viewed on 2 sites – **www.amandasatoz.com** and **http://www.aspenpharma.com.au/atlas/student.htm**

Thank you

Amanda Neill
BSc MSc MBBS PhD FACBS
ISBN 978-1-921930-03-4

T0319294

Table of contents

Abbreviations

A	= actions / movements of a joint	c	= cytoplasm
a	= artery	CD	= cluster of differentiation
aa	= anastomosis (ses)	c.f.	= compared to
AA	= alopecia areata	CFU	= colony forming unit
Ab	= antibody = IL	CIf	= chronic inflammation
Ab/Ag	= antigen antibody complex	CIN	= carcinoma in situ
ABC	= aneurysmal bone cyst	cm	= cell membrane
ACF	= anterior cranial fossa	CMC	= carpometacarpal
AIf	= acute inflammation	CMF	= chondromyxoid fibroma
AIm	= autoimmune	CN	= cranial nerve
adj.	= adjective	CNS	= central nervous system
Ag	= antigen	Co	= collagen
AKA	= also known as	collat.	= collateral
ALL	= anterior longitudinal ligament	CP	= cervical plexus
alt.	= alternative	Cr	= cranial
ANF	= anti nuclear factor	CSF	= colony stimulating factor
ANS	= autonomic nervous system	CT	= connective tissue
ant.	= anterior	D	= dermis / diaphysis
AP	= alkaline phosphatase	Dd	= deep dermis / reticular dermis
A / P	= anterior/posterior	DD	= differential diagnosis
AR	= allergic reaction	DE	= dermo-epidermal junction
art.	= articulation (joint w/o the additional support structures)	diff.	= difference(s)
		DIP	= distal interphalangeal joint
AS	= Alternative Spelling, generally referring to diff. b/n UK & USA	dist.	= distal
		DLE	= discoid lupus erythematosus
assoc.	= associated (with)	DM	= Diabetes Mellitus
B-	= bone marrow derived -	Du	= upper dermis / papillary dermis
B-AP	= bone specific alkaline phosphatase	Dx	= diagnosis / diagnoses
		E	= epiphysis / epidermis
bc	= because	EA	= epidermal appendages
BCC	= basal cell carcinoma	EAM	= external acoustic meatus
BCR	= B-cell antigen receptor	EAS	= external anal sphincter
BM	= bone marrow	EC	= extracellular (outside the cell)
bm	= basement membrane	e.g.	= example
BMD	= bone mineral density	EP	= epiphyseal growth plate
b/n	= between	ER	= extensor retinaculum
br(s)	= branch(es)	er	= endoplasmic reticulum
BS	= blood supply / blood stream	ES	= Ewing's sarcoma
BV	= blood vessel	Ex	= examination
Bx	= biopsy	ext.	= extensor (as in muscle to extend across a joint)
C	= carpal / carpo		

ext.	= extension	LBP	= low back pain generally assoc with prolapsed disc
F	= fat		
f	= fluid	LL	= lower limb
Fab	= antibody binding fragment	lig	= ligament
FB	= fibroblasts	longit.	= longitudinal
FC	= fibrocytes	LOF	= loss of function
Fc	= fragment –crystal region	LP	= low powered magnification
flex.	= flexor	Lt.	= Latin
flex.	= flexion	M	= meta
FR	= flexor retinaculum	m	= muscle
GF	= growth factors	MC	= metacarpal / metacarpo
GH	= growth hormone	MCF	= middle cranial fossa
gld	= gland	MCP	= metacarpophalangeal
GIT	= gastro-intestinal tract	med	= medial
Gk.	= Greek	mito	= mitochondria
grp	= group	MM	= mucous membrane
GS	= ground substance	MNC	= mononuclear cells
H	= hormone	MO	= microorganisms
HA	= hydoxyapatite	MP	= medium magnification
Histo	= Histology	M/P	= medial / lateral
HP	= high powered magnification	MRC	= medical research council
Hx	= history (of the disease)	MT	= metatarsal
IAS	= internal anal sphincter	mΦ	= macrophage
IC	= intercarpal / intercarpo	N (s)	= nerve(s)
If	= inflammation	NA	= nucleic acids
IfR	= inflammatory response / reaction	NAD	= normal (size, shape)
		NAD	= no abnormality detected
Ig	= immunoglobulin	NK	= natural killer
IL	= interleukins = immunoglobulins = Ab	No	= nucleolus
		NOF	= neck of Femur
Im	= immune	NR	= nerve root origin
In	= infection	NS	= nervous supply / nerve system
INF	= interferon	NT	= nervous tissue
inf	= inferior	Nu	= nucleus (nuclei)
IP	= interphalangeal	nv	= neurovascular bundle
IR	= immune response / reaction	OA	= osteoarthritis
Ix	= investigation of	OB	= osteoblasts
ly	= injury	OC	= osteoclasts
jt(s)	= joints = articulations	OG	= osteoprogenitor cells = bone stem cells
l	= lymphatic		
L	= lesion / left	OP	= osteoporosis
lat	= lateral	OS	= osteosarcoma
LB	= long bone	P	= pressure / pus

PAD	=	peripheral arterial / vascular disease
PaNS.	=	parasympathetic nervous system
ParaNs	=	parasympathetic nerves ± fibres
partic	=	particular(ly)
PBM	=	peak bone mass
PCF	=	posterior cranial fossa
PH	=	parathyroid hormone
pH	=	a measure acidity
ph	=	phalangeal / phalanges / phalango
PIP	=	proximal interphalangeal joint
pl.	=	plural
PLL	=	posterior longitudinal ligament
PMNs	=	polymorphonuclear cells = polymorphs
PN	=	peripheral nerve
post.	=	posterior
proc.	=	process
prox.	=	proximal
PS	=	pubic symphysis
PSU	=	pilo-sebacious unit
PVD	=	peripheral vascular disease
Px	=	progress
R	=	right / resistance
RA	=	rheumatoid arthritis
ROM	=	range of movement
RSTL	=	relaxed skin tension lines
RT	=	respiratory tract
S	=	strata/stratum /sacral
SC	=	spinal cord
SCC	=	squamous cell carcinoma
sing.	=	singular
SE	=	side effects
SLE	=	systemic lupus erythematosus
SN	=	spinal nerve
SP	=	spinous process / sacral plexus
SPF	=	sun protection factor
SS	=	signs and symptoms
STL	=	skin tension lines
Su	=	subcutaneous T / fat

subcut.	=	subcutaneous (just under the skin) as a site
sup	=	superior
supf	=	superficial
SyNS	=	sympathetic nervous system
T	=	tissue
TCR	=	T cell receptor
TJC	=	tight junctional complex
Tm	=	tumour(s)
TNF	=	tumour necrosis factor
TP	=	transverse process
Tx	=	treatment / therapy
UL	=	upper limb, arm
v	=	very
V	=	vertebra / vein
VB	=	vertebral body
VC	=	vertebral column
VDRL	=	Venereal Disease Research Laboratory (test for syphilis)
vv	=	visa versa
w	=	with
WBCs	=	white blood cells
w/n	=	within
w/o	=	without
wrt	=	with respect to
&	=	and
∩	=	intersection with
#	=	fracture

Common Terms in Osteology & Pathology

A

Abcess *(AB-sess)* localized collection of pus

Ablation *(AB-lay-shon)* the removal of part of the body, generally a bony part, most commonly the teeth

Achilles (Achilles') tendon AKA Calcaneal tendon, Tendo Calcaneus posterior tendon posterior leg tendon – longest & strongest in the body – 15 cm long up to 4cm wide – joins the posterior muscles to the heel bone

Acro *(AK-roh) (adj acral) Gk akcron = extreme* **end, extremity, peak, tip, denoting something at the extremities ankles / fingers / wrists**

Acromegaly *(AK-roh-meg-al-ee)* adult form of hyperpituitarism – the ends of the long bones continue to grow: coarsen the facial features and digits

Acute *(AK-yewt)* sudden onset + short course – used to describe a condition generally pathological ≠ chronic

Adaptive immunity = Adaptive IR = Aquired IR the response of Ag-specific lymphocytes to Ab, including the development of immunologic memory. Adaptive IRs are distinct from the innate & non-adaptive phases of immunity, which are not mediated by clonal selection of Ag-specific lymphocytes *see also Immunity*

Adnexa *(AD-nex-uh)* appendage, limb extras *pl adnexae (AD- nex-ee)*

Ala *(AY-lar)* a wing, hence a wing-like process as in the Ethmoid bone *pl. - alae.*

Alkaline Phosphatase *(ALK-u-lyn FOS-fat-ayz)* – an enzyme responsible for cleaving the phosphate ion in ATP – ie as a marker of energy consumption – as such it is present on all cells – but specific iso-enzymes may be distinguished – so that bone specific – alkaline phosphatase (B-AP) measures the bone energy activity & is specific to the activity of OBs – bone being formed.

Allergy *(AL-er jee)* abnormal IR to a substance

Alta *Lt. on high* elevation

Alveolus *(AL-vee-oh-lus)* air filled (bone - tooth socket) *adj - alveolar* (as in air filled bone in the maxilla)

Amorphous *(AY-mor-fuss)* shapeless, structure less

Amputation *(AM-pew-tay-shon)* to cut off, to prune, to cut off a limb or appendage

Amyloid *(AM-uh- loyd)* proteinacous substance of varying composition, which appears similar histologically

Amyloidosis – group of diseases characterized by extracellular deposition of the amyloid (3) in Ts & organs – displacing the normal structure e.g. the renal glomerulus (2) or the sinusoids of the liver (4), causing cell & T death (5) & leaving protein casts of their presence (1).

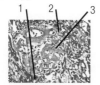
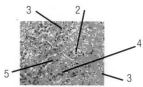

Anaphylaxis *(AN-uh-fill-ax-sis)* exaggerated reaction to a foreign body = acute severe IR

Anatomical position the reference position, in which the subject is standing erect with the feet facing forward, arms are at the sides, & the palms of the hands are facing forward (the thumbs are to the outside).

Anaesthesia loss of sensation

Anatomy *(ah-NAH-to-mee)* the study of the structure of the body.

Ankle bend = angle usually referring to the bend just above the foot, hence the ankle is the joint b/n the foot & LL

aniso   unequal

ankylos – *(an-KEE-los)* **stiff / stiffening – often referring to something becoming calcified**

Ankylosis a fixed bending of the jt – unable to straighten – always pathological

Anlage *(AN – lag) Ger act of laying* = primordium – a clustering of embryonic cells to form an organ or structure

Annulus fibrosis the peripheral fibrous ring around the intervertebral disc

Anteversion – leaning forward

Anthracosis *(AN-thrak-oh-sis)* common benign asymptomatic deposition of carbon (3) in cells macrophages (2) or walled off by fibrosis (4) – generally in lung T (1) but may occur in skin (tattoos)

Antibiotic *(ant-EE-BYE-o-tic)* a substance which can be ingested & used to kill MOs specifically bacteria in the body.

Antibody / Antigen proteins involved in the immune system – antibodies Abs are produced by the body in reaction to antigens Ags proteins or materials found on the surface of foreign bodies introduced to the body forming the antibody-antigen complex

anti– against

Antibodies *see also* **Immunoglobulin** self molecules which are synthesized by the Im cells after being exposed to Ags

Antigen (Ag) usually a foreign macromolecule that triggers the IR & the production of Abs & other immune active molecules e.g. TNF.

Antigen – presenting cells *see Dendritic cells*.

Anti-inflammatory anything which ⬇ If by acting on body responses

Aperture *(a-PET-tyuu-a)* an opening or space b/n bones or w/in a bone.

apo– away from / detached

Apophysis *(APO-fe-sis)* = tuberosity / tubercle cartilage which connects bone to bone or tendon to bone, in young bones (1) but not a true EP (2) – does not function to ⬆ LB length. It is subject to tearing – and separation in overtraining of the young

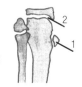

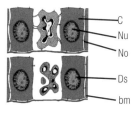

Apoptosis *(a-POP-toe-sis) Gk aptos = to drop out* individual cell death – programmed cell death due to organ conditions – natural cell death – ≠ Necrosis

Appendicular refers to the appendices of the axial i.e. in the skeleton, the limbs upper & lower which hang from the axial skeleton, this also includes the pectoral & pelvic girdles.

Arbor *Gk treelike branches* – arborizing, branching

Areola small, open spaces as in the areolar part of the Maxilla may lead or develop into sinuses.

arth- to do with joints hence…

Arthritis *(AR-thrye-tis)* Inflammation of a joint

Arthrogryposis jt contractures

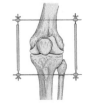

Arthrodesis complete loss of movement in a jt due to surgical ablation – i.e. fusing of the joint – used for pain and loss of mobility – an artificial ankylosis or syndesis

Arthropathy diseases of the joints

Arthroplasty – surgical manipulation of a jt – i.e. its removal or remodeling

Arthrosis AKA arthritis – lower If involvement in the disease process

Articulation joint, description of the bone surfaces joining w/o the supporting structures = point of contact b/n 2 opposing bones hence the articulation of Humerus & Scapula is the articulation of the shoulder joint. *adj articular*

Artifact *(AH-te-fact)* **AS Artefact** – any distortion seen in the histological or radiological processing of material

Atopy *(AY-toe-pee)* – out of place adj atopic

Atrophy *(a-TROH-fee)* *Gk a = lack of, trophe =nourishment* wasting away deterioration of a T or organ from lack of use or food

Atypical not normal, unusual presentation of a phenomenon or structure

auto- (OR-toh)- self

Autoimmune (AIm) pertaining to cells & Abs that arise from & are directed against the individual's own tissues i.e. against "self"

Attrition tooth wear & tear

Atypical *(AY-tip-i-cal)* not usual –often used to describe possible cancerous cells or tissue

audio (OR-dee-oh) pertaining to hearing, or to the ear.

Auditory exostosis = a bony growth on the walls of the EAM (swimmer's ear)

Autolysis (OR-tol-e-sis) – the process of self destruction of a cell or tissue

Autopsy *(OR-top-see)* the examination ± dissection of a body after death – usually to Ix cause of death / verify the diagnosis

Avulsion *(AY-vul-shon)* forcible tearing away of a structure or part of a structure as in an avulsed fracture where a fragment bone is torn away from the main bone

Axis *(AK-sis)* **adj axial** *(AK-see-el)* refers to the head & trunk (VC, Ribs & Sternum) of the body – not arms or legs

B

B cells = B lymphocytes 1 of the 2 major types of lymphocyte. B means the cells come originally from the BM *see also Plasma cells, T cells*

Ball and Socket generally referring to a joint which resembles a ball sitting tightly in a socket - very stable, limited range of movement e.g. hip joint

Basement membrane (bm) a thin layer of extracellular fibrillar protein matrix & CT stroma that underlies all epithelial cells

baso- base (as in acid / base; as in the bottom – the basal layer) *adj basal*

  © A. L. Neill

Basophils – granulocytes of the Im system which take up base staining because of high acid cytoplasmic granules *see also Acidophils, Neutrophils & PMNs*

Basocranium bones of the base of the skull

Basophil *(BAS-oh-fil)* a type of WBC that is characterized by large cytoplasmic granules that stain blue with basic dyes.

Benign *(BEE-nine)* not harmful or dangerous, ≠ malignant, indicating a mild disease. In cancer it is used to describe a mild & non-metastasizing cellular growth.

Biopsy (Bx) *(BY-op-see)* a piece of T removed for microscopic examination – usually from a live person

-blast immature cell / undifferentiated cell

Blount's disease *see Tibia Vara*

Bone *(BOH-n)* a CT that contains a hardened matrix of mineral salts & collagen fibers. Bone cells include: osteoblasts, osteocytes, & osteoclasts.

Bone Mineral Density (BMD) AKA Bone density a score indicating the amount of bone mineral g/cm^2 . It is used as a direct measure of the risk of # and OP. Sites measured are generally high risk # sites of OP – the hip and lumbar spine but any bone is possible to measure. Results are expressed in g/cm^2, note this is not a volumetric measure & so the bone measured is very relevant. T & Z scores determine the type of bone normal osteopenic or osteoporotic

> **T-score,** the number of standard deviations above or below the mean for a healthy 30 year old adult of the same sex & ethnicity as the patient.
> **normal > -1.0 / osteopenia -1.0 to – 2.5 / OP < -2.5**
> **Z- Score,** the number of standard deviations above or below the mean for the patient's age, sex & ethnicity.

Bone spur *see osteophyte*

Boss a smooth round broad eminence - mainly in the frontal bone ♀ > ♂

Bowlegged *see Genu Varus* note there is some confusion here as the term Vargus is also used – but for clarity it is not used here - if this is due to tibial malformation & not a disease of the knee jt per se *see Tibia Vara*

Brachial *(BRAY kee-al)* arm, mainly to do with the upper arm

Bregma refers to a junction of more than 2 bones in a jt as in the Bregma of the skull, junction b/n the coronal & sagittal sutures which in the infant is not closed & can be felt pulsating

Buccal pertaining to the cheek

Bunion *Gk bounion = turnip* abnormal prominence on the inner aspect of the 1st MT head + a bursa & valgus (lat) displacement of the Hallux (big toe)

Bunionette AKA Taylor's bunion enlargement of the lat aspect of the 5th MT head

Bursa *(BER-suh)* a flattened sac containing a film of fluid (B), found around jts to allow for movement. *pl bursae* e.g. the Elbow jt bursa. b/n Humerus (H) & Ulna (U)

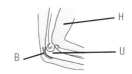

Bursitis If of the bursae

C

Calcaneus *(KAL-kan-ee-us)* heel, hence the bone of the heel *adj calcaneal*.

Calcaneal tendon *see Achilles tendon*

Calcar a spur *adj calcaneal.*

Calcinosis *(KAL-sin-oh-sis)* deposits of Calcium in body Ts &/or organs

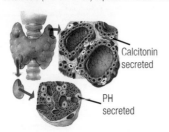

Calcitonin secreted

PH secreted

Calcitonin H secreted by the parafollicular cells of the thyroid gland (1) opposing Ca mobilization – it ⬇ Ca being absorbed in the GIT – being reabsorbed in the renal tubules and being mobilized from bone by ⬇ OC activity, and ⬆ OBs. Its activities are generally not significant as they are over-ridden by PH secreted by the parathyroid gland (2).

Calculus *(KAL-que- lus)* mineral deposit in T **see also stone**

Callus *(KAL-us)* hard T formed in the osteogenic layer of the periosteum as a # repair, replaced over time with compact bone

Calotte *(KALoh-tee)* the Calotte consists of the Calvaria from which the base has been removed.

Calvaria the Calvaria are the bones of the Cranium w/o the facial bones, attached.

Camptodactyly congenital flexion disorder of the PIP, generally affects the little finger

Canal tunnel / extended foramen as in the carotid canal at the base of the skull ***adj canular***

Canaliculus small canal

Cancellous bone = Trabecular bone a spongy, porous bone, lightweight with bone spicules or trabeculae parallel to lines of force found at the ends of LBs (epiphyses) with surrounding BM, found sandwiched b/n lamellae of compact bone, in the VBs & in areas of ⬆ bone thickness

Cancer *(KAN –ser)* group of diseases where the cells w/o the normal controls

Capitulum diminutive of Caput, little head

Capsule *(KAP-syoo-l)* an enclosing membrane

Caput / Kaput the head or of a head, ***adj capitate = having a head (c.f. decapitate)***

Carcinogen *(KAR-sin-oh-jen)* material which leads to cancer formation

Carcinoma *(KAR-sin-oh-mah)* a malignant growth originating from epithelial cells ≠ Sarcoma

Carcinoma – *in situ* pre-invasive cancer still lying in the confines of normal tissue not having broken through the bm but with neoplastic changes

Carpal Tunnel the tunnel formed by the wrist bones (carpal bones) to allow the passage of the flexor tendons & Ns to the hand & fingers, bound superiorly by the palmar fascia

Carpo wrist

Carpometacarpal generally referring to the jt b/n hand & the wrist bones

Cartilage *(KAR-tih-lehj)* a type of CT characterized by the presence of an extensive matrix containing a dense distribution of proteins & a thickened GS.

Caseous *(KAY-zee-us)* cheeselike – a form of necrosis

Cavity *(KAV-it-ee)* an open area or sinus w/in a bone or formed by 2 or more bones *(adj **cavernous**)*, may be used interchangeably with fossa. Cavity tends to be more enclosed fossa a shallower bowl-like space (e.g. Orbital fossa-Orbital cavity).

Cavum a cave *adj cavis*

Cell *(SELL)* the basic living unit of multicellular organisms.

Cephalic pertaining to the head

Cerebral Palsy brain disorder generally from birth or post-In which results in poor muscle control & so leads to bone deformities due to poor coordination & limbs being held in abnormal positions

Cervico- pertaining to the neck

Charcot jt =neuropathic jt

chondro- *(KON-droh)* referring to cartilage

Chondrium *(KON-dree- um)* the cartilage *adj chondria, chondral*

Chondrocyte *(KON-droh-site)* a mature cartilage cell.

Chondrocalcinosis *(KON-droh-kal-sin-oh-sis)* metabolic disorder where calcium deposits are found in jts leading toward their destruction - much like gout with uric acid

Chondroitin sulphate *(kon-DROI-tin SUL-fate)* a semisolid material forming part of the EC matrix in certain CT.

Chondroma *(KON-droh-mah)* benign Tm of cartilage T origin

chromo- *(KROHM-oh)* referring to colour *adj chromatic*

Clinoid like a bed-post, part of a 4-poster bed so that clinoid process looks like a bed post (generally with other posts) as in the Sphenoid bone.

Clavicle little key = S-shaped bone = collar bone

Clivus a slope hence in the ACF referring to a slope on the base of the cavity.

Clones series of cells which are identical to each other; in the IR these are lymphocytes which all produce the same Ags &/or cytokines

Club foot AKA Talipes equinovarus
downward inward pointing foot deformity

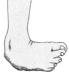

Clusters descriptive term for multiple cells seen to be together but not orientated in any particular manner as opposed to *nests*

Clusters of differentiation (CD) immune cells which express glycoproteins on their surfaces & are seen to act together – specific molecules may be referred to as numbers as in CD4 cells (used to be called leu-3)

Clusters of PMNs used to indicate areas of AI filled with PMNs (neutrophils which have left the BS)

Coagulation *(KOH-ag-you-lay-shon)* process of clotting turning from a liquid to a solid or semi-solid

Cochlea *(KOK-lee-uh)* a snail hence snail-like shape relating to the Organ of Corti in the ear.

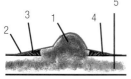

Codman's triangle subperiosteal bone reaction to aggressive bone cancers e.g. osteosarcoma – (1). As the periosteum (2) lifts new bone T forms a triangle (2) b/n the bone & the periosteum via sunray spicules (4). These normal bone spicules develop in reaction to the detached periosteum, from the normal bone (5) underneath not replaced yet by Tm.

Collagen *(KOL-a-jen)* the major fibre of the body; in CT, tendons ligaments & extracellular substances of many Ts

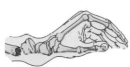

Colles Fracture AKA Colles' fracture # of the distal Radius at the cortico-cancellous junction – looks like a bent fork & sometimes called the fork #. Initially this # excluded Ulna involvement but now this is not always the case & loosely the # may be used to describe any distal forearm #. Common result of falling with an outstretched arm – common # of OP.

Compact bone = Cortical bone = Dense bone bone found in the shafts & on external bone surfaces. The structure is variable & constantly being remodeled throughout life. It may consist of osteons &/or lamellae.

Complement *Lt to fill up or fill out* an entire protein cascade in the BS activated by the presence of bm &/or necrotic cell components, may also be activated in the Ts by allogens – allergic Ag

Complex in IR the combining of 2 factors involved in the IfR or the IR e.g. an Ag & Ab complex which combines to activate or further develop the process

Concha *(KON-kuh)* a shell shaped bone as in the ear or nose *(pl. conchae adj chonchoid)* old term for this turbinate.

Condylar resorption AKA idiopathic condylar resorption process where the condyle of the TMJ is spontaneously resorbed reducing the size of the mandible & affecting the bite – generally seen in adolescent females

Condyle *(KON-dial)* a rounded enlargement or process – used in ref to a number of bones – commonly the TMJ jt

Congenital *(KON-jen-it-al)* present from birth

Connective tissue *(kon-EK-tiv Tish-ew)* (CT) one of the 4 basic types of tissue in the body. It is characterized by an abundance of EC material with relatively few cells & functions in the support & binding of body structures.

Cornu a horn (as in the Hyoid)

Corona a crown. *adj coronary, coronoid or coronal;* hence a coronal plane is parallel to the main arch of a crown which passes from ear to ear *(c.f. coronal suture).*

Cortex the rind or the bark of the tree

Costo/Costa – pertaining to the ribs

Coxa hip

Coxa Plana AKA Perthes disease

Coxa Valga, Norma, Varga with the changing of the femoral angle the Femur exits differently –leading to hip displacement & a limp

Cox algia hip disease

Cranium the cranium of the skull comprises all of the bones of the skull except for the mandible.

Crepitus *(Krep-i-tus)* a grating sensation on jt movement, often present in arthritis; described as bone-on-bone rather than on the articular cartilage

Crest prominent sharp thin ridge of bone formed by the attachment of muscles particularly powerful ones e.g. Temporalis/Sagittal crest

Cribiform / Ethmoid a sieve or bone with small sieve-like holes.

Crown = Vertex the top of the organ or body

Crura *adj cruris* leg

Cuneate /Cuneus a wedge / wedge-shaped (bone)

cyst- *(SIST)* bladder / fluid filled sac

Cyst nodule/tumour filled with liquid semi-solid material lined by epithelium – as opposed to unlined fluid in the **pseudocyst** *adj cystic*

-cytes *(SYTS)* mature cell types

cyto- cellular

Cytokine *(SY-to-kyn)* any substance – generally small proteins made by a cell that affects the behaviour of other cells. Substances made by lymphocytes, act via specific cytokine receptors on the cells that they affect *see also Lymphokines, Interleukins (IL).*

Cytotoxic poisonous to cells – may cause cell death

D

dactyly – digits

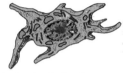

Dendritic (stromal) cells AKA Langerhans cells AKA Antigen presenting cells BM-derived star-shaped/treelike tissue resident phagocytic cells – potent T cell stimulators using Ags attached to stimulate activity, from the monocyte line.

dendro- tree-like formation

Dens a tooth hence dentine & dental relating to teeth, denticulate having tooth-like projections *adj dentate see also odontoid*

Depression a concavity on a surface

Dermatome section of skin (3) supplied by a single NR (2) as opposed to myotome (1) – which is the area of muscle supplied by a single NR – skin & muscle supplied by the same NR are generally closely associated

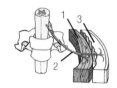

Diaphysis *(DY-af-i-sis)* the shaft or body of a LB. In the young this is the region b/n the growth plates & is composed of compact bone. *pl.= diaphyses adj.= diaphyseal*

Diarthrodal jt = synovial jt = moveable jt

Dislocation when a bone is "out of place" out of its socket – or joint position *see also Subluxation*

Diastasis separation – may mean separation of a muscle from its original position as in pregnancy; or a bone from its original position w/o # – as in tendon rupture

Differentiation the changing of cells to become increasingly specialized

Diploë the cancellous bone b/n the inner & outer tables of the skull, *adj diploic.*

Distal further away from the axial skeleton (opposite of Proximal)

Dolor pain 1 of the 5 cardinal signs of IF

dorsi- back

dys- (DIS) *Gk bad sign* abnormal, bad, difficult, disorganized, painful (opposite to eu)

Dysplasia *(DIS-play-zee-yah)* abnormal growth of T or cells

Dysraphism any spinal abnormality of incomplete closure or malformation including spina bifida

E

Eburnation 2° thickening of the bony end plate (often due to OA)

Edentulous w/o teeth

Effector cells describes those lymphocytes which develop from naïve lymphocytes after initial activation by Ag. They mediate the removal of pathogens from the body w/o further differentiation. Naïve lymphocytes & memory lymphocytes must differentiate &/or proliferate before they become effector lymphocytes.

Effusion excess synovial fluid – in the jt

Elbow any angular bend, e.g.in the UL, referring to the jt b/n the arm & forearm

Eminence a smooth projection or elevation on a bone as in iliopubic eminence.

Enchondroma benign cartilaginous Tm growing on the inside of the bone – surrounded by a bony case – located in the BM, may be a lump of T which never ossified rather than a new cartilage growth **see also chondroma**

Endocranium refers to the interior of the "braincase" *adj endocranial* divided into the 3 major fossae anterior (for the Frontal lobes) middle (containing Temporal lobes) and posterior (for the containment of the Cerebellum).

Endogenous growing from w/in tissues or cells

Endostium a mesodermal CT which lines the inner surface of all bones & is the conduit for the NS & BS of the bone. Lifting of the endosteum causes cancellous bone to be laid down to fill the gap b/n the bone & the cellular layer & this device may be used to encourage bone growth/repair.

Enostosis = boney island a boney growth of compact bone w/in a bone – generally on the internal surface in the trabecular bone harmless incidental finding – DD prostatic metastasis

Epiphysis the end of a LB beyond the growth plate or EP. Generally develops as a 2° ossification centre. There are 2 epiphyses to each LB. Of a LB the shafts are generally compact bone & the ends = epiphyses are trabecular bone with a compact bone covering *pl.= epiphyses adj epiphyseal*

Excrescence outgrowth from a surface – e.g. normal fingernail / abnormal wart or exostosis

Exostosis a bony outgrowth from a bony surface, often due to irritation (as in Swimmer's ear) & may involve ossification of surrounding Ts such as muscles or ligaments.

F

Facet a face, a small bony surface (occlusal facet on the chewing surfaces of the teeth) seen in planar joints.

Falciform *(FAL-see form)* relating to shapes that are in a sickle shape so falciform ligaments curve around & end in a sharp point

Fascia *(FASH-ee-ah) Lt =a band* a sheet or band of fibrous T deep in the skin covering & attaching to deeper tissues

Fascicle *(FAS-ih-kul)* small bundle

Fc receptor the section of the cm which binds the Fc portion of the Ab (IL).

Fever a generalized ⬆ in body temperature due to an ⬆ BF, which may be due to the body's IfR

Femoral angle the angle b/n the femoral head & the shaft   normal 120° – 135°, Valgus >135°, Varus < 120°

Femoral anteversion a leaning forward of the femoral head so that the Femur is rotated & the child becomes knock-kneed ± Patella rotation ± Tibial rotation – developmental rotation which generally spontaneously corrects itself in infancy with re-alignment of the LL – common sitting position is the W – a position preferred by the child.

Fibrino-inflammatory exudates due to IfR with both fibrin & inflammatory components

Fibroblast an immature progenitor cell found in all CT, capable of mitosis, migration, movement. Among other pathways they develop into fibrocytes.

Fibrocyte   mature fibre producing cell = mature **fibroblast** spindle shaped cell producing either collagen (col) or elastin (e) fibres via secretion of monomer units (m) which assemble outside the cell into long fibres, which are then maintained by the fibrocytes. Note with age the number of fibrocytes & hence the fibres ⬇ hence compromising the integrity & strength of their CT. ***See also bone development / structure main text.***

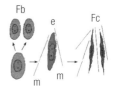

Fibrocartilagenous stroma background T of cartilage with high collagen fibre component

Fibromatosis fibrosis w/n a fascial sheath

Fibrosis *(FY- broh-sis)* ⬆ fibrous T, generally collagen fibres as in scars; can occur in all organs

Fissure a narrow slit or gap from cleft.

Fontanelle a fountain, associated with the palpable pulsation of the brain as in the anterior fontanelle of an infant. These soft spots on the skull are cartilaginous CT coverings "joints" which allow for skull cranial expansion & then become the mould for the bone development & shape joining long the sutural lines, later becoming the Bregma.

Foramen a natural hole in a bone usually for the transmission of BVs &/or Ns. ***pl. foramina***

Fornix an arch

Fossa a pit, depression, or concavity, on a bone, or formed from several bones as in temporomandibular fossa. Shallower & more like a "bowl" than a cavity

Fovea a small pit (usually smaller than a fossa) - as in the fovea of the occlusal surface of the molar tooth.

Fracture (#) = break hence ... ***see main text***

Fusiform spindle-shaped – many CT cells are of this shape particularly fibrocytes.

G

Gallus/Galli a cock, hence, crista galli, the cock's comb *(i.e. possessive form of gallus)*

Gamma Gk letter shaped like a "Y" and used to describe shapes of immunoglobulins

Ganglion a cystic swelling associated with jts &/or tendon synovial sheaths generally on the dorsal surface of the hand or wrist – fibrous capsule containing viscous fluid herniated from the jt /tendon capsule – may press on a N or jt & cause pain

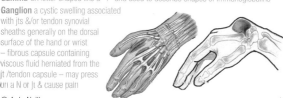

Gene *(JEEN)* a functional unit of heredity that occupies a specific place on a chromosome & directs the formation of a protein.

Genu *(JEN-you)* knee *adj genio* referring to the knee

Genu Recurvatum – hyperextension of the knee jt

Genu Valgus – knock-kneed **("G" knocking together)**

Genu Varus – bow-legged **(AR – AIR in b/n)**

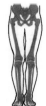 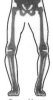 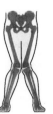

Genu Norma   **Genu Varus**   **Genu Valgus**

Gigantism – overgrowth of the length of the LBs due to excess GH before the fusion of the LBs *see also Acromegaly*

Gomphosis *(GOM-foh-sis)* jt b/n the roots of the teeth & the jaw bones *pl – gomphoses*

Gout *(gowt)* initially a metabolic disorder – accumulation of uric acid crystals in one or several jts – later leading to an arthritis & jt degeneration

Granulocytes cells with granules 2 types in the BS / Immune system - WBCs with granules *see Neutrophils*

Granuloma *(Gran-YOU- low- mah)* a smooth jelly orange-yellow papule nodule which microscopically appears as an aggregation of MNCs; a collection of modified macrophages – epitheloid cells, histiocytes surrounded by lymphocytes ± GCs & fibrocytes – attempting to wall off the area from the surrounding T, a granuloma is a feature of Clf *see also Granulomatosis*

Granulomatosis – the process of forming granulomae a response in Clf when there is no resolution of the process.

Groove long pit or furrow

Ground substance AKA Extrafibrillar matrix – refers to the material in T which is not fibrous or cellular & found outside the cells – v prominent in all CTs.

Growth factors natural substances produced by the body or obtained from food that promote growth & development by directing cell maturation & differentiation and by mediating maintenance & repair of Ts.

H

Haemarthrosis blood in the jt cavity

haemo *(HEEM-oh)* **AS hemo-** referring to blood

Hallux the big toe = the first toe

Hamus a hook hence the term used for bones which "hook around other bones or where other structures are able to attach by hooking - hamulus = a small hook.

Harris lines AKA growth arrest lines lines of ⬆ bone density due to pathological assault or sudden growth spurts. They indicate the position of the EP at the time of the event but they may change the shape of the bone & affect its length. Only seen in Xrays

Haversian canals = osteons *see Osteons*

Heberden's nodes OA of the DIP of the hand resulting in swellings & deformities of the jt

Heterotopic ossification formation of bone outside the skeleton – occurs around jt replacement – partic the hip, #s & after paralysis, ectopic bone forms & immobilizes the jt – graded by the amount of movement limitation, progresses until the jt is immobilized - Grade IV no mobility.

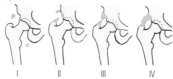

| I | II | III | IV |

Hinge joint jt with movement in one plane e.g. elbow or knee

Histamine vasoactive amine stored in mast-cell granules – basophilic histiocytes

histio-/hist-/histeo *Gk histos = web* tissues

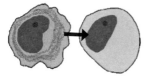

Histiocyte *(hist-EE-oh-site) Gk histio- tissue = phagocytic tissue cell* a cell in the tissues which is immunologically active, derived from the BM mononuclear line. In CIf they may undergo epithelioid transformation *see also Granulomatosis*

Hormone *Gk hormaein = to spur on* a substance secreted in the body having a regulatory affect on organs & Ts

Hyaline *Gk – glassy* smooth glassy generally refers to hyaline cartilage found on the surface of synovial jts to facilitate movement of the 2 bones over each other; but may indicate T changes in which the T takes on a glassy – hyaline appearance

Hydroxyapetite = Hydoxlapatite, (HA) = **bone mineral**, is a naturally occurring mineral form of calcium apatite $Ca_5(PO_4)_3(OH)$, but is usually written $Ca_{10}(PO_4)_6(OH)_2$ to denote there are 2 entities. The OH^- can be replaced by: carbonate, chloride or fluoride as in fluridated water. Up to 50% of bone by weight is a modified form of hydroxylapatite.

Hyoid U-shaped

Hyperostosis abnormal bone growth, thickening, generally overgrowth or ectopic growth

Hyperthyroidism condition of an overactive thyroid gland which may affect the bone and cause OP *see also Thyroid hormone & Calcitonin*

hypo- underneath / below

Hypoxia *(Hy- poks-ee-uh)* – lack of Oxygen but not the absence of it ≠ anoxia

I

Ideopathic of unknown origin

Immune *(IM-youn) Lt – immunis = to free, to exempt* free from the possibility of acquiring a certain disease or infection

Immune Complexes Ab/Ag combinations used to stimulate the IR

Immune response (IR) any response made by an organism to defend itself against pathogens.

Immune system a coordinated system of cells, T & soluble products that constitutes the body's defense against invasion by non-self entities, e.g. infectious & inert agents & tumour cells.

Immunity a state of biological defense using an entire system of cells, structures & substances – immune system – to combat infectious agents or biological invasion, in either a non-specific (innate immunity) or specific way (adaptive immunity).

Immunoglobulins (Ig) = antibodies Ab proteins involved in the IR either secreted or fixed on the cell surface

Immunology the study of the cell, tissues, organs & substances involved in the body's defense against attack by microbes, foreign bodies or tumours, & any adverse consequences of the IR *see also Inflammation.*

Incisura a notch.

Inclusion any foreign or heterogeneous substance w/in a cell not introduced as a result of trauma.

Infarct *(in-FARK-t)* death of cells or Ts due to coagulative necrosis – death of T due to blockage of the BS

Inferior under

Inflammation = Inflammatory Response (IfR) the body's stereotypical response to damage indicated by 5 cardinal signs: dolor = pain; calor = heat; tumor = swelling; rubor = redness; function laesa = loss of function

  acute (AIf) immediate, severe, short lived, predominant cells PMNs

  chronic (CIf) slow onset, long lasting, associated with long term irritation & healing, predominant cell types MNCs   note chronic may or may not be an extension of the acute inflammatory process

Inter between

Interleukins *(inter-LOO-kins) (IL)* "communication b/n leucocytes" *see also Lymphokines* often designated IL-X with X a number indicating specific characteristics of the signals instigated by this IL

Intra within

Intracellular inside the cell

Introitus *(in-TROY-tus)* an orifice or point of entry to a cavity or space.

Involucrum bone formed via the periosteum when lifted as in purulent osteomyelitis

J
Joint = Articulation + supporting structures

K
Knock-kneed *see Genu Valgus*

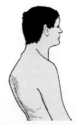

Kyphosis *(KYE-foh-sis)* collapse of VBs causing sharp convexity of the spine – in the thoracic region (note due to the lumbar curve it is rare to see an absolute convexity in the lumbar region & a kyphosis will often exaggerate the lumbar lordosis)

L

Lacerum something lacerated, mangled or torn e.g. foramen lacerum small sharp hole at the base of the skull - often ripping T in trauma.

Lacrimal related to tears & tear drops. **(noun lacrima)**

Lambda Gk letter a capital 'L' - written as an inverted V. **(adj lambdoid)** – used to name the point of connection b/n 3 skull bones Occipital and L & R Temporal bones.

Lamina a plate as in the lamina of the vertebra a plate of bone connecting the vertical & transverse spines **(adj lamellar, pl. laminae)** e.g. **lamellar bone** layers of compact bone interdigitated with sheets of collagen fibres these may form concentric rings around BVs as in osteons (Haversian systems) or as layers around the outside & inside of the diaphysis of LBs

Lamina dura layer of immature bone lining the tooth socket

Lesion any single area of altered tissue or part of an organ

leuco-/ leuko- AKA luco /luko *(LOO- koh)* **white, pale, clear**

Leucocyte *see* **white blood cell (WBC)**

Ligament (s) a band of CT which connects bones (articular ligaments) (1) or viscera - organs (visceral ligaments), generally collagen A ligament is a tie or a connection. Originally it was used as sing. **ligamentum pl ligamenta** from ligate or to tie up generally composed of collagen fibres. **see also Tendons** (2)

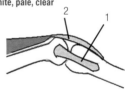

Linea a line as in the Nuchal lines of the Occiputum / Occipital bone

Lingus *(ling-GUS)* tongue **adj Lingual** *(ling-GEW-al)* pertaining to the tongue

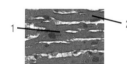

Lipofuscin *(LIE-poh-fus-kin)* "brown fat" is actually a protein (1) indicating aging or severe stress in a cell; ⬆ with age; seen commonly in muscle (2) & skin cells but may be present in any cell

Lipping bone projecting over the usual margin, excessive production generally pathological as in OA, may interfere with jt movement

Locus *(LOH-kus)* a place **(c.f. location, locate, dislocate)** – specific area in organ or T of either cell division or specialization

Looser's zones AKA pseudofractures opposite of Harris lines, horizontal lucent lines or areas seen in the X rays indicating regions of inadequate of mineralization occurring in bone growth or remodelling seen in osteomalacia

Lordosis *(lor-DOH-sis)* concavity in the VC – cervical & lumbar region have this normal curve which may become exaggerated – predisposes to LBP **opposite to kyphosis**

-lucent *(LOO-sent)* **transparent, clear**

-lymph *(LIM-pf)* **clear liquid**

Lymphatic – a vessel which carries fluid – lymph - to the heart

Lymphocytes small round single nucleated WBCs derived from the BM or the thymus gld, one of the MNC types, which produce Abs & are involved in the IR **see also B cells, T cells and main text – BM**

Lymphokines Cytokines made by lymphocytes. **see also Cytokines, Interleukins.** All lymphokines are cytokines but not vv

Lysosomes toxic cellular organelles containing enzymes which digest material – if lysed thoy will dcstroy their host cell

M

macro- big, large

Macrodactyly overgrowth of one or more digits

Macrophage *(MAK-roh-farj)* (mΦ) Tissue MNC, originally from the BM to the BS & then migrated out to the T.

Magnum large *pl magna*

Major histocompatibility complex (MHC) found on cells to determine self & non-self

Class I = found on all nucleated cells & present to Cytotoxic T cells

Class II found on certain immune cells B cells / Macrophages / dendritic cells – present to

Helper T cells

Malignant process which is rapid disconnected & uncontrolled as opposed to benign – so a malignant growth will be rapid & metastasize.

Malleus hammer (as in the ear ossicle)

Mandible from the verb to chew, hence, the movable lower jaw; *adj mandibular.*

Mast cells large cells found in CTs throughout the body, most abundantly in the submucosal tissues & the dermis. They contain large granules which play a crucial role in allergic reactions.

Mastoid breast or teat shape - mastoid process of the Temporal bone.

Maxilla the jaw-bone; now used only for the upper jaw; *adj maxillary.*

Meatus a short passage; *adj meatal* as in EAM connecting the outer ear with the middle ear.

Meniscus *Gk. crescent* – relating to the cartilaginous intra-articular crescents in the knee jt

Mentum relating to the chin (mentum = chin not mens = mind) *adj mental.*

Meta an extension of...: cf. metacarpal = extension of the wrist

Metacarpophalangeal (MCP AKA MP) generally referring to the jt b/n hand & finger

Metaphysis = Epiphysis the slightly expanded end of the shaft of a bone.

Metaplasia the changing of one form of T type to another, extending from one type to another type as it grows

Micronutrient similar to trace element but it includes any substance which is essential to the body's normal functioning but is only needed in minute amounts. Deficiencies are rare in most cases because the dietary needs are so low; they often involve bone metabolism. Common micronutrients are: Aluminum, Boron, Chromium, Copper, Fluoride, Manganese, Molybdenum, Silicon, Zinc

Monocytes WBCs with a large single bean-shaped nucleus, part of the MNCs group. Monocytes that leave the BS are called macrophages & those residing in the T are histiocytes.

morph- *(MORF-)* shape / form

Mucus *(MEW-kus)* slippery gelatinous substance produced by mucoid glands AKA phlegm *adj mucous also mucoid* – mucus-like & myxoid *(MIKS-oyd)* generally referring to substances found in Tms which have a mucus-like appearance slimy & jelly – in these cases it is pathological

Multiforme *see also* **Polymorphic**

myco- *(MY-coh)* **relating to fungi**

myelo- *(MY-loh)* **to do with the BM or the SC**

Myelocyte *(MY-loh-site)* – young cell in the WBC granulocyte series, may go on to become Acidophil, Basophil or Neutrophil.

Myotome section of muscle (1) supplied by a single NR (2) as opposed to dermatome (3) – which is the area of skin supplied by a single NR – skin & muscle supplied by the same NR are generally closely associated

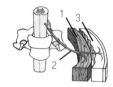

N

Necrolysis death of cells due to liquefaction

Necrosis *(NEK-roh-sis)* pathological cell death due to hydrolytic proteins & causing an IfR reaction as opposed to **Apoptosis** differences b/n them are:

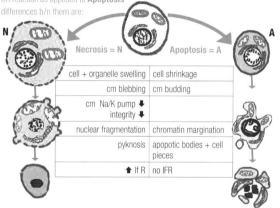

Necrosis = N	Apoptosis = A
cell + organelle swelling	cell shrinkage
cm blebbing	cm budding
cm Na/K pump ⬇ integrity ⬇	
nuclear fragmentation	chromatin margination
pyknosis	apopotic bodies + cell pieces
⬆ If R	no IFR

Neoplasia *(NEE-oh-play-zee-yuh)* **Gk neo = new, plasia = growth** any uncontrolled growth which may metastasize & spread directly or indirectly in an uncontrolled or poorly controlled manner often losing many or all specialized features of their original tissue *adj neoplastic see also Benign*

Nests descriptive term for multiple cells orientated circularly & growing into the centre of the circle as opposed to cells with no particular orientation – *clusters*

Neurocranium the neurocranium refers only to the braincase of the skull.

Neuroma benign proliferation of neural T but is often used to denote a fibrosis / fibrous nodule particularly in the feet as in plantar *neuroma*

Neutrophils *AKA Granulocytes* – WBCs with granular cytoplasm of neutral staining histologically & multi-lobed nuclei. When these migrate from the BS they are called polymorpho-nuclear cells (PMNs).

Nigricans darkening, a lesion which shows ⬆ brown/black pigment

noci- *(NOH-see)* **pain**

Notch an indentation in the margin of a structure.

Nucha *(NEW-kuh)* the nape or back of the neck adj.- nuchal.

Nucleus *(NEW-klee-us)* nut – brain of the cell containing DNA

Nucleolus *(NEW-klee OH-lus)* brain w/n the brain – nub of DNA material inside the nucleus

O

Occiput the prominent convexity of the back of the head Occipitum = Occipital bone *adj occipital*

Occulus an eye

Odontoid relating to teeth, tooth like ***see Dens***

Ontogeny the development of an individual growth pattern

Orbit a circle; the name given to the bony socket in which the eyeball rotates; *adj orbital.*

Orifice an opening.

Orthosis general bone disease

occulta **hidden**

Oedema AS Edema *(uh-DEEM-uh)* swollen *adj oedematous*

-oid **like / similar to**

-ology **study of**

-oma **lump / tumour**

Omo *(OH-moh)* shoulder

Ontogeny the development of an individual growth pattern

Organelles – small intracellular structures e.g. mitochondria

Orifice an opening.

ortho- **straight**

Orthosis AKA orthotic device
device to correct the movement of a bone or bones – from the simple foot orthoses to complex neck braces - the study of which device to use or make is the study of orthotics *pl. orthoses*

Os a bone or pertaining to bones *adj osseus*

Ossicle a small bone as in the ear ossicles: Stapes (stirrup), Incus (anvil) & Malleus (hammer).

-osis **disease of – non-inflammatory – implying a degeneration**

Ossification the process of turning into bone. Normally this is confined to bony T & occurs in 2 ways - but in cases of hypercalcaemia & other conditions this may occur pathologically, ossifying parenchyma.

Osteitis *(OS-tee-eye-tis)* Inflammation of the bone

Osteoarthritis AKA degenerative arthritis low inflammatory disease of the joints - due to a wearing away of the cartilage & exposure of the subchondral bone

Osteoarthrosis similar condition to the previous entry but w/o inflammation – these 2 terms are often used interchangeably - differentiated mainly in discussions on the TMJ

Osteoblasts immature bone cells – capable of dividing & laying down matrix

Osteochondritis *(os-TEE-oh-kon-dry-it is)* If of the articular bone & cartilage – leading to disintegration of the bone & then cartilage in the jt (osteochondritis dissecans) - often due to poor BS with avascular necrosis the underlying cause

Osteochondritis Dissecans deterioration of the subchondral bone and hence cartilage from lack of BS, "dessicating " the jt. Generally affects the larger jts – hip, knee, shoulder, often of young boys (10-18yo).

Osteochondroma *(os-TEE-oh-kon-DROH-muh)* – benign bone & cartilaginous Tm often arising in the EP which protrudes at right angles, common & asymptomatic

Osteochondrosis a familial group of diseases where there is focal disturbance of enchondral ossification – i.e. the bone may be poor in original formation or degenerate to cartilage – seen in the VC of adolescents

Osteoclasts = Giant Cells used interchangeably multinuclear cells which resorb or phagocytose bone.

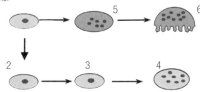

Related to macrophage & the MNCs in the following way – a common haemopoetic stem cell (1) under stimulation – & site will differentiate into a monocyte (2) then macrophage (3) & when stimulated by foreign bodies into giant cells (4) much as in remodeling of bone – the cells for pre-osteoclasts (5) which become activated under hormonal & other influences into osteoclasts (6)

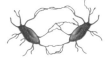

Osteocytes mature bone cells, incapable of dividing but maintain the extracellular matrix of the bone – they interconnect through a series of cytoplasmic canaliculi through the calcified matrix

Osteogenesis formation & growth of bone, from scratch

Osteoid uncalcified bone / bone-like

Osteoma Tm of the bone T

Osteomalacia disease of softening of the bones / Paget's disease

Osteomyelitis inflammatory disease of the bone due to In

Osteons (AS osteones) = Haversian systems the system of concentric circles of compact bone &collagen fibres surrounding the central BVs, & Ns (1) – a with other systems via perforating BVs – or Volkmann canals (2).

Osteophyte *(o-STEE-oh-fite)* AKA bone spur bone overgrowth or spike – generally pathological due to If damage to the T. Normal cartilage (1) is often eroded leaving bare damaged bone (2) which stimulates a new bone growth – osteophyte (3). They also occur at the site of ligament & tendon insertion particularly in the

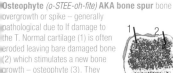

VC as in shown in the Xray & MRSA images of the lumbar spine (4).

The A to Z of Bone & Joint Failure

Osteoporosis AKA smooth bone atrophy a thinning of the bones due to an imbalance b/n remodeling & new bone formation & / or calcium deficiency. Both cortical & cancellous bone is diminished & the bone weaker, often unable to withstand normal forces resulting in pathological #s.

Osteosarcoma malignant Tm of bone T

Osteosclerosis an ⬆ density of bone often due to compression #s or a reaction to avascular necrosis or other If processes – detected on the X-ray.

Osteotomy realignment of a jt by cutting through the adjacent bone

Ostium *(o-STEE-um)* a door, an opening, an orifice.

Otic pertaining to the ear

Ovale oval shaped

P

Palate: a roof *adj palatal or palatine.*

Pallisading – term used to describe cells usually epithelial/epitheloid forming in lines like a fence around or along a structure

Pannus AKA Granulation Tissue abnormal layer of fibrovascular T associated with chronic If – found in jts with RA, on the cornea & other areas. It contains If cells & substances –e.g. macrophages & interleukins which grow eroding & destroying the underlying T. It is always pathological.

para- Gk to one side

Paratendinitis If changes w/n the tendon sheath

Parietal pertaining to the outer wall of a cavity; from paries = a wall.

Parotid pertaining to a region beside or near the ear

Pars a part of

Patella kneecap

Patella Alta a condition where the kneecap (1) sits abnormally high (2). It contributes to patellofemoral instability, early OA, pain in the knee & is either congenital or due to constant quadriceps contraction as in ballet pointe work or the wearing of high heels in early adolescence – opposite to **Patella Baja** (AKA Patella Infero) (3), which is commonly seen after surgery on the knee, particularly knee jt replacement.

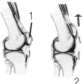
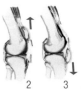

Pathogenesis the origin or cause of the pathology of a disease.

Pathogens MOs / substances that can cause disease when they infect/invade a host.

Pathognomonic applied to a symptom which if present indicate conclusively a specific disease

Pathophysiology the part of the science of disease concerned with disordered function as distinguished from physical defects.

-pathy disease of

Pedis *(PED-is)* pertaining to feet

-penia *(PEEN-ee-yuh)* **lack of**

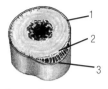

Perforating fibres AKA Sharpey's fibres
collagen fibres perforating through the periosteum (1) to connect & bind ligaments, tendons & the periosteum to the bone T (2). These collagen fibres (3) if lifted will stimulate the formation of new bone.

peri- around

Perikymata transverse ridges & the grooves on the surfaces of teeth

Perivascular surrounding BVs generally capillaries

Perikymata transverse ridges & the grooves on the surfaces of teeth

Periosteum layer of fascial tissue CT on the outside of compact bone not present on articular (joint) surfaces *see endosteum*

Periostitis inflammation on the outer surface of the bone

Periostosis abnormal growth of LBs on their outer surfaces

Pes any part of the LL below the ankle – generally refers to the foot

Petrous pertaining to a rock / rocky / stony *adj petrosal*

phaeo- *(FAY-oh)* **brown dusky**

phago- *(FAY-goh)* **to eat / eater**

Phagocyte any cell that can ingest/eat bacteria, foreign particles, &/or other cells.

Phalanx pertaining to flanks of soldiers - phalanges a row of soldiers used for a row of fingers or toes *adj phalangeal as in interphalangeal jts see metacarophalangeal jts*

-phil *(FILL)* **lover of**

Phlegmon *(FLEG-mon)* unconfined If – as opposed to **Abscess** confined If

-phobe *(FOBE)* **hater of**

Phytates *(FYE-tates)* the salt form of phytic acid = the major form of phosphates in plants & grains – it chelates many cations & interferes with their absorption – including Ca & Mg, but also Fe, Zn. It is a large 3 dimensional cage-like molecule with a central hexagonal carbon ring surrounded by PO anions. It attracts metal cations in the digestive system & ⬇ their absorption.

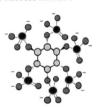

Planar joints jt which allows for sliding across the jt as in the wrist, foot & ribs

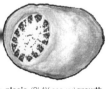

Plasma cells – derived from B cells are large Ab producing cells with central clock-faced nuclei

-plasia *(PLAY-see-yu)* **growth**

-pluri- **multiple**

Pluripotent description of a substance / cell which has the ability to develop in many different ways e.g. stem cells are pluripotent.

-podia *(POH-dee-yu)* **pertaining to feet (often the formation of feet for cell movement)**

poikilo- *(POYK-il-oh)* **spotted, mottled, irregular**

Poliomyelitis *(POH-lee-oh-my-e-lye-tis)* upper motor neurone disease resulting from viral In – leading to cerebral palsy – **see cerebral palsy**

poly- many

Polydactyly extra digits – congenital

Polymorphic many shaped **see also Multiformc**

Pollex thumb

Process a general term describing any marked projection or prominence as in the mandibular process.

Pro-inflammatory cytokines family of cytokines that promote If. e.g. TNF = tumor necrosis factor

Prominens a projection

Proximal closer to the axial skeleton (opposite of distal)

pseudo *(SEW-doh)* **false**

Pseudoarthrosis false or new jt due to the non-healing of a #

Pseudogout see chondrocalcinosis

Pterion *(TERY-on)* a wing; the region where the tip of the greater wing of the sphenoid meets or is close to the parietal, separating the frontal from the squamous region of the Temporal bone **adj pterygoid .** alternatively the region where these 4 bones meet.

Pubis hairy – that part of the hip bone with hair over the surface **adj pubic pl. pubes**

Pus yellow/white creamy discharge associated with the IfR representing necrotic T **adj purulent** *(PEW-roo-lent)* pus forming

Pyarthrosis *(PIE-ar-throh-sis)* pus in a jt space

Pyknosis *(PIK-noh-sis)* shrinking of the nucleus in a cell – generally pathological

pyo- *(PYE-oh)* **Gk pus**

pyogenic = suppurative pus forming

Q

Q angle AKA quadriceps angle the angle made b/n the quadriceps insertion & the tibial line – similar to the tibiofemoral angle, used to determine genu vargus & varus – draw a line from the ASIS to the centre of the Patella – then from the Tibia to the ground 6° NAD > 6° knock knees; < 6° bow legs

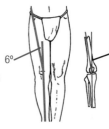

R

Rachitic *(RAK-it-ik)* description of the uncalcified osteochondroid mixture observed in rickets – & Vitamin D deficiencies

Ramus branch as in the superior pubic ramus the superior or higher branch of the pubic bone (Pubis)

RANKL = Receptor activator of nuclear factor kappa-B ligand is a cytokine belonging to the TNF (tumour necrosis factor) group, specifically related to bone metabolism. It is a surface bound molecule found on OBs which activates OCs to start resorbing bone. It has other roles in the immune & calcium metabolism system.

Reactive Arthritis a 2° arthritic reaction which may occur after an In this may take place weeks - months after the initial triggering event generally an infection

© A. L. Neil

Recess a secluded area or pocket; a small cavity set apart from a main cavity.

Rectus *(REK-tus)* **AKA ortho** straight – erect

recte- straight *adj recticular*

Reduction the return of a bone or joint to its proper place after dislocation &/or subluxation

Re-modelling the forming & reforming of bone in its normal growth cycle

Reiter's syndrome reactive arthritis after a bacterial infection – MOs lodging in jts randomly also associated with skin diseases

Rickets form of osteomalacia or bone softening due to Vitamin D deficiency

Ridge elevated bony growth often roughened.

Rotundum round

S

Sarcoid *(SAR-koyd)* **Gk sarc -flesh** see also **Granulomas**

Sarcoidosis a disease in which "sarcoid deposits " resembling granulomas are placed in various organs in the body including in 25% of cases the skin. In the skin the disease is self limiting, but the disease may resolve spontaneously or continue and prove fatal it is difficult to Dx & treat. Aetiology idiopathic *see also Granulomatosis*

Sarcoma – Gk fleshy lump malignant tumour derived from cells of mesenchymal (CT) origin

Sagittal an arrow, the sagittal suture is notched posteriorly, making it look like an arrow by the lambdoid sutures.

Sclerosis hard / hardening *(adj sclerotic)*

Scoliosis *(SKOH-lee-oh-sis)* abnormal lateral curvature of the VC

Scurvy – Lt Scorbitus = ascorbic acid adj scorbutic

AKA Barlow's disease when in infants

> *Presentation* red non-blanchable skin spots, easy bruising, poor wound healing, malaise & lethargy, bone pain, bleeding gums & loose teeth
>
> *Aetiology* deficiency in Vitamin C
>
> *Pathogenesis* the inability to stabilize collagen which is constantly turned over and needed in skin, MM & all CT maintenance & wound healing

see also Diseases of Micronutrient deficiency – Beriberi, Pellagra

Sella a saddle; *adj sellar*, sella turcica = Turkish saddle.

Sequestrum *(SEE-kwes – strum)* devascularized bone fragments – as in osteomyelitis & fractures *pl sequestra*

Sesamoid grainlike

Sharpey's fibres *see Perforating fibres*

Sigmoid S-shaped, from the letter Sigma which is S in Greek.

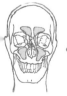
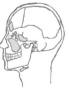

Sinus a space usually w/n a bone lined with MM, such as the frontal & maxillary sinuses in the head. Sinuses may contain air, venous or arterial blood, lymph or serous fluid depending upon location & health of the subject *adj sinusoid.* also, a modified BV usually vein with an enlarged lumen for blood storage & containing no or little muscle in its wall; as in the brain venous sinuses

Skull the skull refers to all of the bones that comprise the head.

Spheno- *(SFVEE-noh)* a wedge i.e. the Sphenoid is the bone which wedges in the base of the skull b/n the unpaired Frontal & Occipital bones *adj sphenoid.*

Spina Bifida congenital failure of the closure of the posterior processes of the vertebral canal

Spine a thorn *adj spinous* descriptive of a sharp, slender process / protrusion.

Splanchocranium the facial bones of the skull.

spondy- to do with the vertebra, or vertebral column

Spondylitis degenerative OA of the VC – associated with back pain due to the lf processes & impingement on the NR outlet

Spondylolysis malformation or deterioration of the pars articularis the jts b/n the vertebrae – presents with back pain

Spondylosis *(SPON-dee-loh-sis)* degeneration of the VC – often used to describe back pain – but this use is incorrect

Spondylosis Deformans ankylosing of VBs by growth & extension of osteophytes along the VC

Spongiosis intercellular oedema - reversible T damage in the early stages

Squamous flat, square-shaped

Steatosis fatty change reversible cell damage accumulating fat intracellularly

Stress Fractures overuse injuries - # which occur through constant low mechanical force as in jogging or running – or any repetitive activity on weight bearing areas – this may also occur in weakened bones, particularly in OP & Paget's disease. Sites of stress fractures in normal bones –
(1) cracks in the lower leg bones – & their epiphyses
(2) but they occur in the feet & toes particularly with dancers (3, 4). The fractures are multiple, superficial & repair with rest and cessation of the activity if possible – Common sites: Ankle, Heel, Humerus, Metatarsals, Tibia, & VC

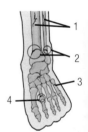

Stroma background T which may be fibrillar with occasional resident cells present, or matrix & extracellular material, in a T, GS & the assoc. cells present which do not represent the main T or organ

Subchondral – beneath cartilage – generally referring to the bone just below the articular cartilage

Subluxation displacement of bones / joints – when a bone is out of place, partially or completely dislocated, used a lot in chiropractic to describe the partial mal-alignment of the vertebrae & their joints *see also Dislocation*

Sulcus long wide groove often due to a BV indentation

Sustenaculum a supportive structure as in the sustenaculum tali = a structure which supports the Talus in the foot

Suture the saw-like edge of a cranial bone that serves as jt b/n bones of the skull.

Stylos an instrument for writing hence *adj styloid* a pencil-like structure.

Symphysis a cartilagenous joint or a growth with bone-cartilage-bone

syn- means together i.e. the close proximity of, or fusion of 2 structures

Syndactuly *(SIN-dak-til-ee)* congenital condition where digits are fused together

Syndesmosis tight inflexible joints b/n 2 bones little to no movement as in many axial jts

Synostosis fusion of any joints

Synovectomy removal of the synovial membrane generally done in RA to minimize jt damage

Synovial joint = Diarthrosis any moveable joint with synovial fluid b/n the 2 opposing bones – most moving joints are synovial. *See main text*

Synovitis If of the synovial membrane *see also Tenosynovitis*

Systemic *(SIS-tem-ik)* involving the whole body

T

T cells = T lymphocytes 1 of the 2 major types of lymphocyte. These cells have sub groups but all are derived from the thymus. Reduction in these numbers results in ⬇ immune protection & excess may cause Alm diseases.

T-score *see bone mineral density*

Talipes *(TAL-i-pez)* a twisted foot

this is used in various combinations derived from the foot's normal movements

   1 dorsi flexed – **talipes equines**

   2 plantar flexed – **talipes calcaneus**

   3 abducted & everted – talipes valgus

   4 adducted & inverted – **talipes varus**

   including combinations of these descriptions or abnormal bone shapes

   5 high instep – **talipes cavus**

 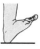

   1   2   3   4   5

Talus *(TAY-lus)* ankle **(Gk. bend)**

Tarsus pertaining to any bones joining the foot with the leg *adj tarsal* (*Gk wickerwork* referring to the basketlike structure of the os tarsus with the ligaments)

taxis locomotor movement of cells

Tectum a roof.

Tegmen a covering.

Temporal refers to time & the fact that grey hair (marking the passage of time) often appears first at the site of the Temporalis.

Tendinitis AS Tendonitis Alf of the tendon, degeneration may result & deterioration to tendinosis

Tendinopathy general term incorporating many of the pathological changes which may occur in the tendon

Tendinosis degeneration of the collagen fibres w/n the tendon w/o inflammatory cells

It is often difficult to distinguish b/n bone & tendon disease – the key is to see if the site of the tenderness moves when the joint moves (tendinosis – b) or remains fixed (bone pain – a).

endo Calcaneus anatomical name for Achilles tendon – *see also Calcaneal tendon*

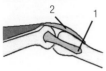

Tendon (1) a tie or cord of collagen fibres connecting muscle with bone (as opposed to articular ligaments (2) which connect bone with bone)

Tenosynovitis Alf of the synovial capsule & the tendon which is passing through it – a combination of tendinitis + synovitis

Tentorium a tent.

Thrombocyte AKA Platelet – small piece of a megakaryocyte which circulates in the B to plug up any damage in the BVs & stimulate the clotting process

Thyrocalcitonin AKA Calcitonin see Calcitonin

Thyroid Hormone H secreted by the follicular cells of the thyroid gland does not in the \normal thyroid affect the bone metabolism but in hyperthyroidism – this H ⬆ levels of serum Ca – mobilizing it from the bone via the OCs & so may hasten or cause OP **see also Calcitonin**

Tibia Vara AKA Blount's disease – abnormal growth of the medial tibial plateau – resulting in exaggerated bow-legs

Tibiofemoral angle see also Q angle the angle b/n the Femoral shaft & the Tibia

Tophus (TOH-fus) deposit of uric acid crystals due to gout

Trabecula a "little" beam i.e. supporting structure or strut **pl. trabeculae**

Trace elements similar to micronutrients but it is to be noted a lot of trace elements have a low range of effectiveness & if present in excess are toxic. **see also Micronutrients**

Trephination the practice of making an artificial hole in the cranium practiced in many ancient religions used to relieve cranial pressure

Trochanter pertaining to a small wheel or disc in the femur it is a large disc shaped tuberosity

Trochlea a pulley, that part of the bone or ligamentous attachment that pulls the bone in another direction as in the elbow or the ankle

Tubercle a small process or bump, an eminence.

Tuberculum a very small prominence, process or bump.

Tuberosity a large rounded process or eminence, a swelling or large rough prominence often associated with a tendon or ligament attachment.

Tumour AS Tumor lump, swelling

Tumour Necrosis factor (TNF) family of cytokines first implicated in cancers causing cell death, known to be involved in the IfR

U

Uncus a hook **adj. uncinate.**

Ureotelic ability to get rid of urea from the system

V

*Valgus AKA Valga L knock kneed, twisted bent out = away from the midline describes an increase in the angle of the distal portion of the bone, used to describe the angle b/n the femoral head & shaft – the femoral angle, the carrying angle of the arm & the tilt of the hip or angle of the foot

Varus AKA Vargus AKA Vara *L bow legged* describes a decrease in the angle of the distal part of the bone

* there is a great deal of confusion in the use of these terms bc of the origin as described above – so a valgus knee is knock-kneed but so is a varus hip   so common usage with knees has come to be – **VALGUS KNEE = knees knocked together (A)** & **VARUS KNEE = knees with air in b/n (B).**

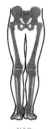 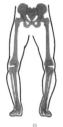 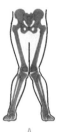

NAD   B   A

Vertex – top, superior point

Volkmann's canal = perforating canal connecting channels in compact bone b/n osteons & perforating the lamellae of the osteon & bringing in the periosteal lining

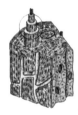

W

White blood cells (WBC) = leucocytes general term for all blood borne cells which appear white on the blood smear / BM smear - includes: monocytes, lymphocytes & granulocytes

Wormian bone extrasutural bone in the skull

X

Xanthoma *(ZAN-thoh-muh)* deposition of cholesterol subcutaneously or may be located in the tendon – tendon xanthoma

Z

Z-score *see bone mineral density*

Zygoma a yoke, hence, the bone joining the Frontal, Maxillary, Sphenoid & Temporal bones *adj zygomatic.*

Structure of Bone Tissue

Bone is a tissue. It contains osteocytes (mature bone cells -1), osteoblasts (new bone cells -2), osteoclasts (resident monocytes) which may combine to form GIANT cells aka osteoclasts (3) to remodel bone which occurs constantly.

The tissue may be packaged as COMPACT bone – dense bone for major weight-bearing areas as in the Long bones or as CANCELLOUS bone = spongy bone = trabecular bone, which is present in the axial skeleton and at the heads of most Long bones.

The density of bone is changing all the time. It is one of the most dynamic tissues in the body constantly forming and reforming its structure. Its repair capacity is extensive, but changes in body demands, diet and disease states will affect its integrity.

> **Loss of bone = Osteoporosis**
> **Excess deposition of bone = Osteopetrosis**
> **Deposition of bone in ectopic sites = Ossification**

COMPACT BONE – A

It is surrounded by an outer fascial layer – Periosteum (4) and an inner fascial layer – Endostium (5) and has a central cavity filled with Bone Marrow (BM) – either filled with fat cells – YELLOW BM – or haemopoietic tissue (cells related to forming the blood and its component cells) – RED BM. The bone is laid down in circular layers or lamellae (6L) with a central core (6c) for the BS, called HAVERSION systems (7).

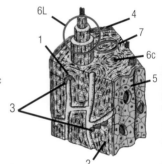

CANCELLOUS BONE – B

This consists of long trabeculae or spicules of bone laid along pressure lines surrounded by haemopoietic tissue – RED BM (8). It is highly mobile; the first to be mobilized for mineral needs or changing body function, and gives support to the compact bone. This may result in a weakening of this load bearing bone and haemorrage into the area along with fractures (9).

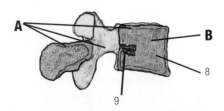

Classification of Bones

FLAT BONES are thin, flattened and curved, e.g.: most Skull bones, Scapulae, Manubrium & Sternum They are generally surrounded by a layer of compact bone with cancellous or spongy bone in b/n.

IRREGULAR BONES have various shapes not easily classified: Ear, Clavicle, Hip, Rib, Sphenoid bones & Vertebrae. They have irregular growth centres.

LONG BONES These bones are long with a shaft = diaphysis and 2 ends epiphyses. They have growth centres at each end and grow lengthwise over years via their growth plates at the metaphyses, e.g.: most limb bones: Femur, Fibula, Humerus, Radius, Tibia, Ulna, & digits Phalanges, see Diagram.

PNEUMATIC BONE/ALVEOLAR BONES are filled with air to lighten their weight, e.g.: Maxilla, Frontal, Mandible, Ethmoid. These vary from small airpockets to large sinuses.

SESAMOID BONES are completely surrounded by soft tissue w/o joints e.g.: Hyoid, small bones around the thumb and big toe.

SHORT BONES are roughly cubic in shape. e.g.: most wrist = Carpal, ankle = Tarsal bones and many of the bones at the base of the skull.

SUTURAL BONES = "Wormian" bones are small bones which occur w/in the skull sutures. They are sometimes called extra-sutural if the main part f the bone is outside of the suture. They are unnamed, except the Incus – the largest extra-sutural bone.

There are: 22 paired skull bones including the ear ossicles/ not including the teeth.

5 single bones mainly on the base of the skull

1 mandible

1 hyoid

variable sutural and extra-sutural bones (generally between 3-5)

There are 56 digit bones or Phalanges plus an additional 3 to 4 small sesamoid bones in the foot over the big toe and the thumb

Each limb has a single long bone proximally (arm = HUMERUS, & thigh = FEMUR), an hinge joint (ELBOW & ANKLE) and 2 bones distally (the forearm = RADIUS & ULNA and lower leg (shin) = TIBIA & FIBULA) joined by an interosseous upper membrane – ligament made up of strong CT.

Each pair of limbs is supported by a GIRDLE of supporting bones; the PECTORAL GIRDLE = the SHOULDER GIRDLE and the PELVIC GIRDLE = the HIP GIRDLE.

There are b/n 600 and 620 bones in the human body.

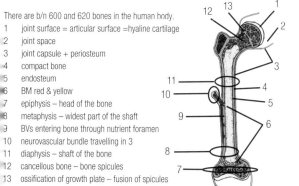

1   joint surface = articular surface =hyaline cartilage

2   joint space

3   joint capsule + periosteum

4   compact bone

5   endosteum

6   BM red & yellow

7   epiphysis – head of the bone

8   metaphysis – widest part of the shaft

9   BVs entering bone through nutrient foramen

10   neurovascular bundle travelling in 3

11   diaphysis – shaft of the bone

12   cancellous bone – bone spicules

13   ossification of growth plate – fusion of spicules

The Cell – overview

Micro Schema – Most cells contain organelles – internal structural components which maintain the homeostasis and life – variations occur depending upon the specialization-differentiation – and current function of the cell. A lack of/or fault with any of these components may lead to metabolic disease states and/or other pathologies.

1   2 centrioles – involved in the cell's aging

2   microvilli – outpouchings of the cm – devices to the surface area of the cell

3   microfilaments, intermediate filaments and microtubules – giving structure to the cell

4   peroxisome – involved in cellular defence and digestion

5   mitochondrion – 2X layered rod-shaped organelle – involved in the production of the cell's energy

6   membrane pores – allowing passage of materials in and out

7   lysosomes – used to destroy material in the cell

8   endoplasmic reticulum (er) – used for intra cellular communication

   r = rough er i.e. ribosomes attached (rer)
   s = smooth w/o ribosomes (ser)

9   cellular waste products extruded via secretory vesicles

10 nucleolus (No)

11 nucleus (Nu)

12 nuclear membrane and pores

13 Golgi apparatus – produces cm

14 cytoplasmic blebs

15 ribosomes – involved in protein synthesis

16 cytoplasm – GS of the cell

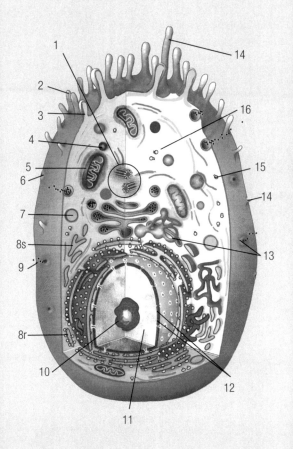

Bone Tissue - cellular components

Micro Schema – Bone T is one form of CT – derived from the embryological 2nd layer – the mesenchyme. Like all CT the cells may develop in many ways. The following schema demonstrates some of these pathways. Note the extensive matrix around these cells.

1   fibroblasts (FB) mature to fibrocytes (FC) – which maintain the collagen fibres and GS of many Ts e.g. the dermis / loose CT = areolar T as well as tendons and ligs.

2   stimulated fibrocytes (FC) may return to the more immature state of the FB so that they may multiply (mitosis), for e.g. after ly – to form scar T etc.

3   FB may differentiate into chondroblasts (CB), then chondrocytes (CC) which maintain the extensive GS of cartilage.

4   # & intermembranous bone formation cause FBs to differentiate directly to osteoblasts (OB) and form bone.

5   CB further differentiate into bone in EP of LBs – endochondrial ossification

FB are active mitosing cells, containing more organelles than FC. OB divide regularly but do not produce as much GS as the OC. OB also divide and may become lining cells of the endosteum or periosteum or coalesce and become osteoclasts, as well as mature bone cells.

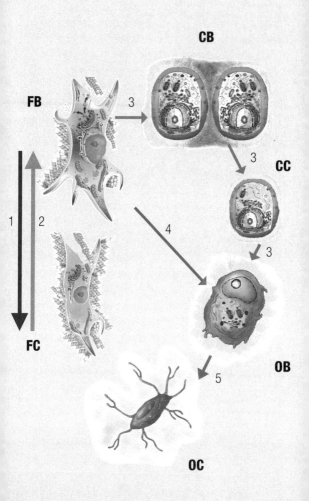

CB

FB   3

3   CC

1   2

4

3

FC

OB

5

OC

Bone Marrow – cell types

In childhood nearly all the BM is red, the site of haematopoiesis – this changes with development and in the adult the red BM is confined for the most part in the BM of the axial skeleton. Starting from a pluripotent stem cell (S) several different cell types develop via predestined pathways. These then move to the BS and in some cases out to the T, particularly in response to injury and/or inflammation.

E erythropoietic cell line – leading to the erythrocyte (RBC) in the BS pro-erythroblasts (1) become erythroblasts (2, 3, 4) – losing their DNA completely as reticulocytes (5) before being released to the BS as mature erythrocytes (RBC) (6).

G granulocytes derived from the myeloid line develop into myeloblasts (1) and then pro-myelocytes (2) before further differentiating into the granular leucocytes which have multilobed nuclei and their intracellular granules have different staining affinities: basophils (3) neutrophils (4) or acidophils (5).

L lymphoid cell lines develop in the BM as lymphoblasts (1) which further differentiate (via pro-lymphocytes -2) finally into lymphocytes (3) which may directly leave the BM – B lymphocytes or go to the thymus – T lymphocytes.

M monocytes (2) – so-called because of their single nucleus and agranular cytoplasm develop from monoblasts (1)

P platelets (3) develop from the cytoplasmic pieces of the megakaryocytes (2) – huge cells which develop from megakaryoblasts (1) which reside in the BM

Some of these BM derived cells move out of the BS to the Ts and either reside there permanently or are induced to go there under If influences. In the Ts these take on new names and new properties, with specific roles in the IfR.

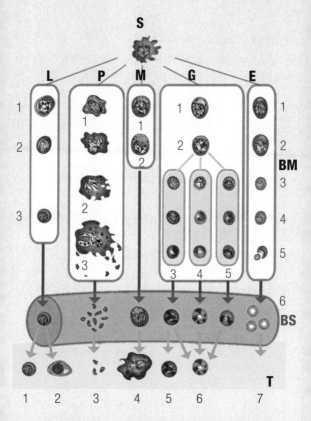

1 B or T lymphocytes =
  B or T cells

2 plasma cells – from B cells

3 platelets clot outside the BS

4 macrophage / histiocyte
  – may coalesce to form
  multinucleated giant cells

5 mast cells

6 polymorphonuclear cells
  (PMNs)

7 RBCs extravascularly
  become clots

Bone Marrow – cell types
Red BM – tissue in situ

In childhood nearly all he BM is red, the site of haematopoiesis – this changes with development & in the adult the red BM is confined for the most part in the BM of the axial skeleton. Starting from a pluripotent stem cell lines form several different cell types through predestined pathways. These then move to the BS & in some cases out to the T, particularly in response to injury &/or inflammation.

The red BM changes slowly to yellow BM as the fat cells replace the haemopoietic T with the lengthening of the bones.

1 adipose = fat cell & nucleus

2 sinusoid capillary to allow cells to pass through into the BS

3 stroma – reticular T

4 arteriole =a / venule =v

5 myelocytes

6 megakaryocyte

7 pro-myelocyte

8 neutrophilic myelocytes

9 eosinophilic myelocytes

10 erythroblasts

11 normoblasts

12 erythrocytes

13 reticular cells – part of the CT of the BM

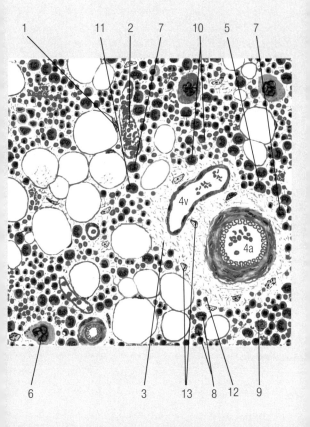

Bone Development – Intermembranous Ossification

Flat and Irregular bones

Bones of the skull and other irregular bones do not develop from a cartilage anlage, but rather from the mesenchymal T itself by direct ossification. This is less flexible in that it is harder for these bones to change length and shape with age.

A   mesenchyme (HP)

B   condensed mesenchymal cells undergoing proliferation

C   osteogenic progenitor cells (OGs) forming calcified matrix in the GS – osteoid

D   woven bone – islands with osteoblasts (OBs) and osteocytes calcified GS with large gaps in b/n forming BM – highly vascularised later forming outer plates of compact bone (MP)

E   remodelling end stage (LP) skull – diploë

1   mesenchymal cell (stem cell)

2   capillary

3   fibroblast

4   CT ground substance loose areolar T

5   fibrocyte

6   OGs

7   mitosis

8   OB

9   calcified GS

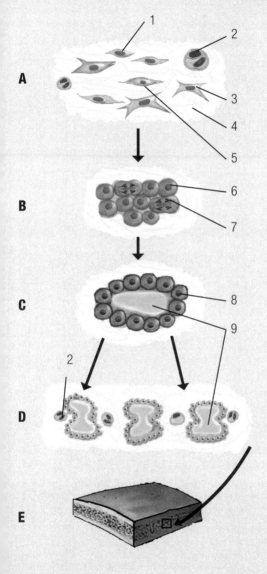

Bone Development –
Intermembranous Ossification
Developing Skull

The skull develops via intramembranous ossification

The skin (1) lies over the vascular CT (2) which contains the BVs and Ns (3) of the region, and is continuous with the forming periosteum (4). The periosteum at this stage is continuous with the BM cavities (5). Bone trabeculae (6) contain OBs (7) surround the BM cavities which contain primitive CT (8) and their BVs (9). Collagen fibres (10) travel from the periosteum to the trabeculae and the adjacent BM cavities. OBs deposit osteoid – the newly synthesized bone matrix (11) around the developing trabeculae which contains OCs (12) in their lacunae they form mature bone matrix (13). Even at this stage bone re-modelling is occurring using the giant cells (osteoclasts) (14) while other areas are quiescent with little activity. Fibroblasts in the CT (15) may transform into OBs directly and go on to form more bone T.

Schema – Histo (MP) section of developing intramembranous bone development in the skull

 1 skin
 2 primitive CT
 3 BVs and Ns of CT
 4 periosteum
 5 BM cavities
 6 bone trabeculae
 7 osteoblasts = OBs
 8 CT
 9 BVs
10 collagen fibres
11 osteoid – primitive bone matrix
12 osteocytes = OCs in their "holes" – lacunae
13 mature bone matrix
14 giant cells = osteoclasts
15 fibroblasts

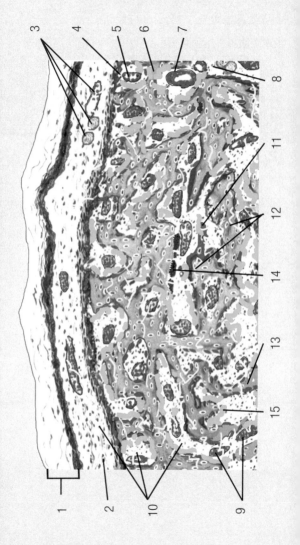

Bone Development – Endochondrial Ossification

Long Bone (LBs)

Most bones of the appendicular skeleton are LBs. After the condensation of the mesenchymal CT they develop and form a cartilage anlage, the model of the bone to develop. Length is able to continue after the main bone formation via EPs.

A   Mesenchymal condensation forming cartilage anlage

B   Chondrocytes stimulated to grow

C   Osteogenic metaplasia

D   Bone cells attracting BS – cartilage has no BS

1   CT

2   chondrocytes

3   hypertrophic chondrocytes

4   osteoblasts – forming a bone collar

5   BVs

6   perichondrium

7   10 ossification centre + BM

8   periosteum

9   compact bone

10   20 ossification centre + BS

11   bone spicules

12   endosteum

13   EP

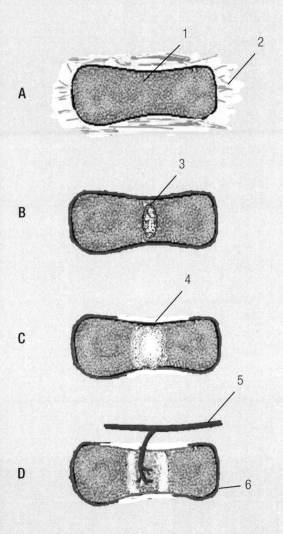

A

B

C

D

Bone Development – Endochondral Ossification

Long Bone (LBs)

Most bones of the appendicular skeleton are LBs. After the condensation of the mesenchymal CT they develop and form a cartilage anlage, the model of the bone to develop. Length is able to continue after the main bone formation via EPs.

E BM formation

F increased LB length

G Diaphysis elongation

H Epiphyseal ossification EP formation

1 CT

2 chondrocytes

3 hypertrophic chondrocytes

4 osteoblasts – forming a bone collar

5 BVs

6 perichondrium

7 10 ossification centre + BM

8 periosteum

9 compact bone

10 20 ossification centre + BS

11 bone spicules

12 endosteum

13 EP

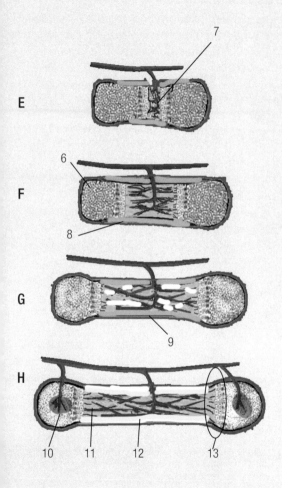

E

7

F

6

8

G

9

H

10 11 12 13

Bone Fracture – Healing Process
Long Bone (LBs) – simple break

The principles of fracture repair are similar in all fractures – there is a response to the broken and dead T. B in the area forms a clot and then stimulates cells and substances to respond in a pre-determined fashion. Altogether the bone is one of the most dynamic Ts in the body with extensive regenerative/repair capacity, to the extent that 2 years after the repair of an uncomplicated fracture, the new bone T is indistinguishable from its surroundings.

Haematoma formation

1   compact bone
2   medullary cavity – site of BM
3   lacerated BVs
4   clot = haematoma + fibrin + cellular components
5   periosteum lifted due to bleeding into area
6   bone fragments

Callus formation 2-3 weeks

7   collagen fibres – Sharpey's fibres were ripped on the lifting of the periosteum – stimulating new fibre synthesis
8   fibroblasts – mobilized by the clot & the lifting of the periosteum
9   pro-callus formation – woven bone + dead bone pieces
10 dead bone
11 new capillaries drawn into the area

Callus ossification
4 weeks –< 2 months (depends upon the extent of the #)

12 proliferating OB
13 trabeculae of forming bone – compact bone
14 reconnection of the BS throughout the bone T
15 fibrocartilagenous callus remnants

Remodelling – ongoing

16 re-organized bone – along lines of stress
17 OC – multinucleated phagocytes involved in bone re-modelling
18 Re-establishment of the medullary cavity – and BM

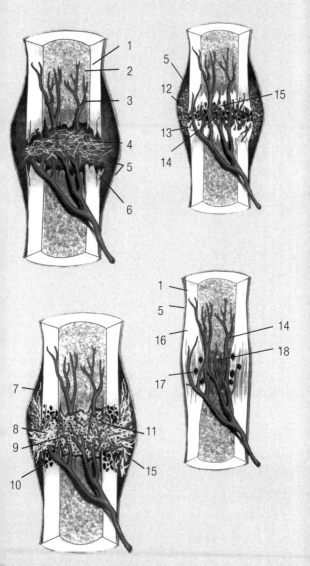

Fracture Classification – Fracture Types
Long Bone (LBs) – simple break
Fractures are described according to:

> *their position – and whether the break is exposed or not*
> *the direction of the break*
> *the type of break*

Position

1 proximal

2 midshaft

3 distal

4 simple – i.e. closed = # not exposed

5 compound i.e. open – # is open = pierced through the skin

Direction

6 longitudinal

7 oblique

8 spiral

9 transverse

Type

10 avulsed = a segment of bone is pulled away

11 butterfly = a piece of bone chipped out from the main bone

12 comminuted = small pieces of bone in the #

13 impacted = the bone is "squashed" due to the # – generally because of powerful muscle contraction

14 incomplete = greenstick – generally with young bones – which are not fully ossified

15 pathological – generally due to a weakening of the bone from neoplasia and/or atrophy (as in OP)

16 segmental = a single large piece of bone separates from the main #

Note that site specific fractures are also described – e.g. Bennett's fracture (of the thumb) – these relate to the specific difficulties of these particular #s – for example peculiarities of their BS etc but they can also always be classified using the described schema

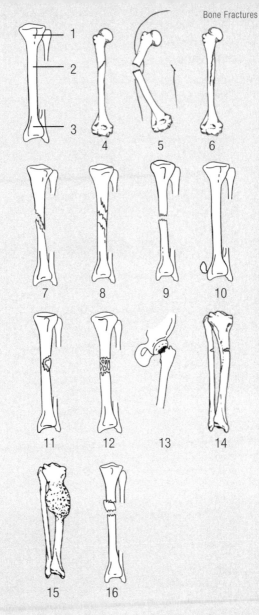

Lower Limb alignment –
normal development

LL development follows a typical predictable pattern due to the in utero position of the leg – the following stages occur in the LL development

infants – gentle Varus – bow-leg

< 2yo – the lower leg is nearly straight

3-4yo – a Valgus develops – knock kneed

> 7yo – the Valgus reduces – and this is maintained throughout life

1 in utero – note the bowing of the LLs
2 4 months
3 18 months
4 3 ½ yo
5 7 yo

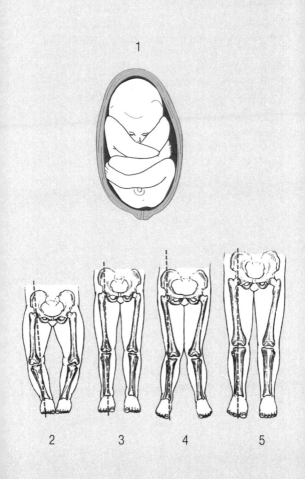

Bone Age - Skeletal Maturation
Stages of Ossification

The Bone Age – *is the degree of skeletal maturation, which commences with the appearance and development of ossification centres in the embryonic tissue. This differs b/n bones, ethnic origins and sex. Males generally mature later than females. 1° and 2° ossification centres appear w/n the CT framework (onset of the maturation process) and continue to expand until they fuse at puberty i.e. completely mature. This occurs over a time range demonstrated in the following tables/graphs, which shows some bones demonstrating greater variation than others. Growth (increase in length and mass) is a related but separate process. Both may be retarded by nutritional deficiencies and febrile chronic illnesses and altered by congenital abnormalities of the adrenal, pituitary and thyroid glands and ovaries and/or testes.*

The time of the ossification determines the site of fractures in immature bones as EPs are weaker than formed bone. EPs are also the first area to show the effects of factors which influence bone growth and development, altering the subsequent rate and type of ossification.

Hand & Wrist Development

The hand develops over a number of years – first the cartilage anlage develops ossification centres which become EPs then the wrist bones undergo ossification and the MCs; finally the LBs of the forearm and fingers.

3 images – schema relating changes in the 5yo hand, 8 yo hand & 17yo hand

1　Phalanges / finger bones
2　Metacarpals (MCs) / hand bones
3　Carpal bones / wrist bones
4　Radius
5　Ulna
6　Epiphyseal growth plates (EPs)

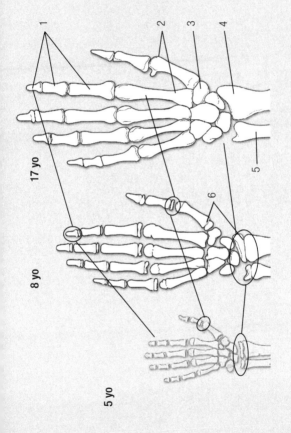

1

2
3
4

17 yo

5

6

8 yo

5 yo

Elbow

Solid ossification

red = ♀

blue = ♂

Dotted fusion v

red = ♀

blue = ♂

Epiphyseal growth plates

1 med. head of the Humerus
2 lat. head of the Humerus
3 Capitulum of the Humerus
4 Trochlea of the Humerus
5 head of the Radius
6 Olecranon of the Ulna

A **fusion of the Humerus**
B **fusion of the Radius**
C **fusion of the Ulna**

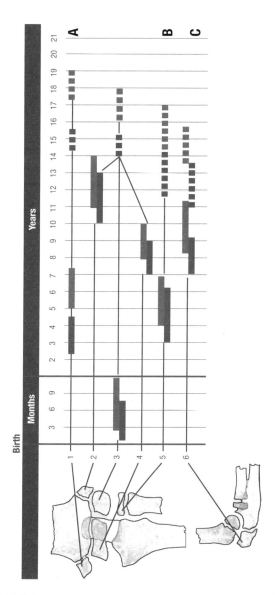

Foot and Ankle

Solid ossification	■■■■ red = ♀
	■■■■ blue = ♂
Dotted fusion v	■ ■ ■ ■ red = ♀
	■ ■ ■ ■ blue = ♂

Epiphyseal growth plates ▬▬▬▬

1 distal epiphysis of the Tibia
2 medial malleous (Tibia)
3 dist. epiphysis of the Fibula = lat. malleous
4 epiphysis of the Calcaneus
5 Calcaneus main body (present from birth)
6 Talus (present from birth)
7 Navicular bone
8 Cuboid (present from birth)
9 Medial Cuneiform = 1st cuneiform
10 Intermediate Cuneiform = 2nd cuneiform
11 Lateral Cuneiform = 3rd cuneiform (present from birth)
12 MT epiphyses

A fusion of the Tibia
B fusion of the Fibula
C fusion of the Calcaneus
D fusion of the MTs – medial 1st through to the lateral

Note the Phalanges – toes – follow the MT fusion

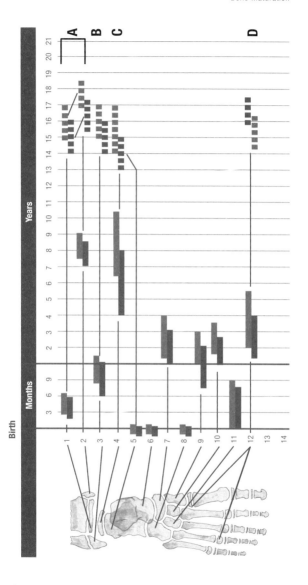

Hand and Wrist

Solid ossification   ▬▬▬ red = ♀

                                  ▬▬▬ blue = ♂

Dotted fusion v   ▬ ▬ ▬ red – ♀

                                  ▬ ▬ ▬ blue = ♂

Epiphyseal growth plates   ▬▬▬

1. phalangeal epiphyses – fingers
2. MC epiphyses 2-5
3. Hamate
4. Capitate
5. 1st Sesamoid bone of the Thumb
6. Trapezoid
7. 1st MC epiphysis
8. Trapezium
9. Triquetral
10. Scaphoid
11. Lunate
12. Pisiform
13. distal epiphysis of the Radius
14. distal epiphysis of the Ulna

A   fusion of the finger bones – distal 1st and proximal last

B   fusion of the hand bones – MCs through from the 2nd to the 5th

C   fusion of the Radial and Ulna epiphyseal plates

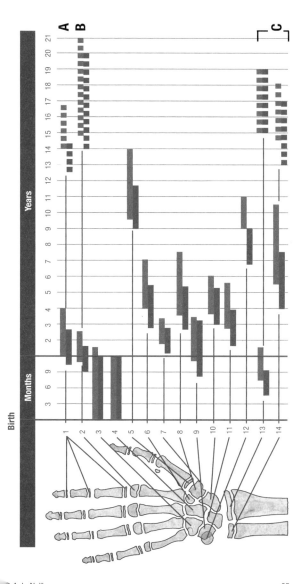

Hip Joint

Solid ossification

red = ♀
blue = ♂

Dotted fusion v

red = ♀
blue = ♂

Epiphyseal growth plates

1   crest of the Ileum
2   acetabulum – note is the fusion of 3 bones
    Ileum / Pubis & Ischium which make up the hip
3   Ischium and Pubis
4   Ischial tuberosity
5   apophysis of the Pubis
6   head of the Femur
7   greater trochanter of the Femur
8   lesser trochanter of the Femur

A   fusion of the hip bones
B   fusion of the Femur

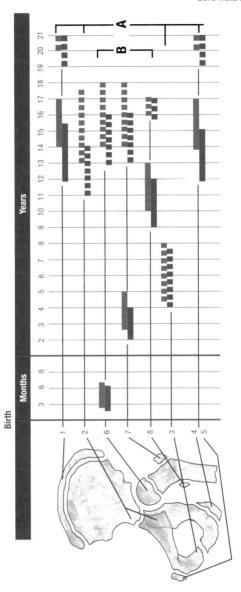

Knee Joint

Solid ossification ███████ red = ♀

███████ blue = ♂

Dotted fusion v ▬ ▬ ▬ ▬ red – ♀

▬ ▬ ▬ ▬ blue = ♂

Epiphyseal growth plates ░░░░░░░

1 dist. epiphysis of the Femur (present at birth)
2 Patella
3 prox. epiphysis of the Tibia (present at birth)
4 Tibial tuberosity
5 prox. epiphysis of the Fibula

A fusion of the Femur epiphyseal growth plates
B fusion of the Fibula epiphyseal growth plates
C fusion of the Tibia epiphyseal growth plates

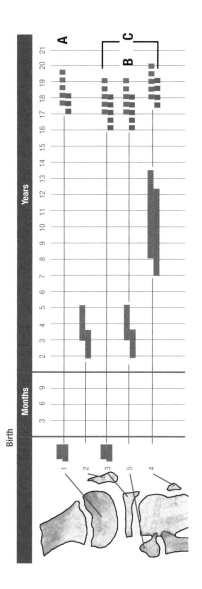

Shoulder Joint

Solid ossification

████████ red = ♀

████████ blue = ♂ ♂

Dotted fusion v

▬ ▬ ▬ ▬ red = ⚲

▬ ▬ ▬ ▬ blue = ♂

Epiphyseal growth plates

1   head of the Humerus
2   greater tubercle of the Humerus
3   medial end of the Clavicle

A   fusion of the head and greater tubercle
B   fusion to the Humeral shaft
C   fusion of the Clavicle (last jt to fuse in the body –
    after 20s)

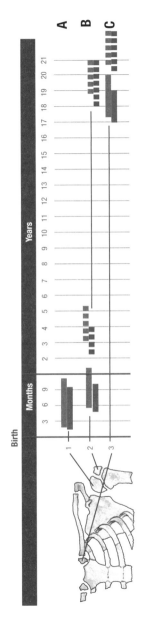

Bone Structure
Cancellous bone – Vertebra

The Skull develops via intramembranous ossification

The vertebra is made up of cancellous (trabecular bone) with a thin outer layer of compact bone as do most of the bones of the axial skeleton.

Dense CT (1) surrounds the bone which merges with the periosteum (2), which is attached to the thin layers of compact bone (3) and the forming trabeculae (4) which surround the BM cavities (5) & their BVs. All inner surfaces are lined with the endosteum – composed of fibroblasts (6) which may develop into OBs (7) and form bone under stimulation.

Although these bones do not have as many osteons (8) as in the bone shafts of LBs – they exist and are constantly forming (9) and re-forming due to bone's constant re-modelling. They are composed of OCs and their lacunae (10). The enclosed red BM is highly vascular and contains haemopoetic T (11)

Schema – Histo (MP) section of cancellous bone – vertebral body

1 CT
2 periosteum
3 compact bone
4 trabecula
5 BM cavities
6 fibroblasts
7 osteoblasts = OBs
8 osteon
9 forming osteon – developing – or re-forming
10 osteocytes = OCs in their "holes" – lacunae
11 haemopoetic T

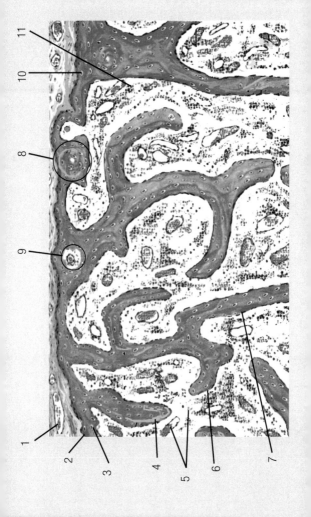

Bone Structure
Long Bone (LBs)

Macro Schema – *Most LBs have an outer compact bone shell and inner spongy – cancellous bone which is thin in the bone shaft – diaphysis but present throughout the ends – epiphyses. The central core is BM – either yellow predominantly fat, or red – predominantly haemopoetic (blood forming) T. This schema shows the LB structure.*

1   joint surface articular surface hyaline cartilage
2   joint capsule
3   joint capsule continuous with the periosteum – contains NS and BS of the bone
4   outer – compact bone
5   endosteum – inner lining of the bone – contains BS and NS of the bone
6   BM – red and yellow
7   epiphysis – head of the LB
8   metaphysis – widest part of the bone shaft
9   BVs entering the bone through nutrient foramen
10 neurovascular bundle entering into the bone via the periosteum
11 diaphysis = bone shaft
12 cancellous bone = trabecular bone = spongy bone
13 ossified EP = originally cartilagenous growth plate – ossification prevents further the bone becoming longer

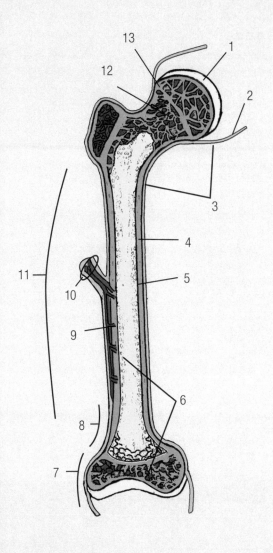

13

1

12

2

3

4

5

11

10

9

6

8

7

Bone Structure
Long Bone (LBs)

Micro Schema – Most LBs have an outer compact bone shell and inner spongy bone which is thin in the bone shaft – diaphysis but present throughout the ends – epiphyses. The central core is BM. This schema shows a cross section through the shaft of a LB.

1 outer lamellar circumferential system

2 osteon = Haversian system

3 cement line – b/n osteons – calcified GS

4 central BV

5 collagen fibres – helical with alternate directional turns in each layer of the osteon

6 inner lamellar circumferential system

7 spicule of spongy bone = trabecular bone = cancellous bone

8 spicules connect with each other along the force lines of the bone

9 BM

10 endosteum – lines inner bone surfaces – contains OG cells

11 BVs + central canal of the osteon

12 OC

13 Volkmann's canal – perforating osteon lamellae

14 periosteal space + inner periosteal layer

15 Sharpey's fibres – collagen fibres connecting to the bone T

16 periosteum – containing BS to the bone

17 interstitial lamellar bone – remnants of old remodelled osteons

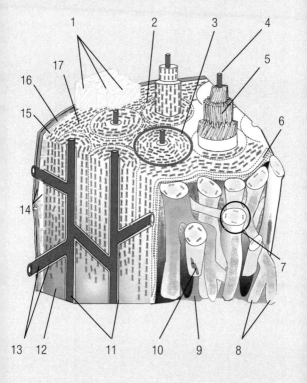

Bone Matrix - Mineralization

OBs secrete matrix vesicles which are dispersed through the collagen fibres of the CT

These then attract more calcium ions and become more mineralized, until the matrix becomes a solid calcified ground substance – osteoid.

Schema – CT ground substance to Osteoid matrix

A   zone A – newly formed matrix vesicles

B   zone B – early mineralization of the GS

C   zone C – increasing deposition of the minerals into the GS

D   zone D – confluent mineralization

E   zone E – early mineralized bone

1   OB

2   matrix vesicles

3   collagen fibres

4   mineralized material – attaching to vesicles

5   confluence of solid matrix

6   complete solid GS – basis of mature bone matrix – after re-modelling

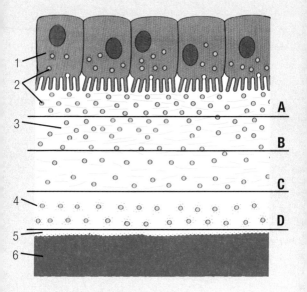

1

2

3

A

B

4

C

5

D

6

Bone – Remodelling
Causes – force changes

With changed forces – bone will be stimulated to change its shape & to increase its size (w/in limits) with Increased weight bearing. These processes may occur together as well as sequentially, dependent upon the force directions and sizes.

Schema – Bone with altered directional force & amount

A   New Force - stimulating bone re-modelling

B   re-modelling

C   model shape complete

D   new bone - cannot determine where the old bone was

E   thickened bone – due to increased force

1   new force direction

2   increased weight bearing force

3   area possible for the re-modelling

4   new bone – note direction of bone in line with the force internally

5   old bone resorbed – because it is outside the main force line

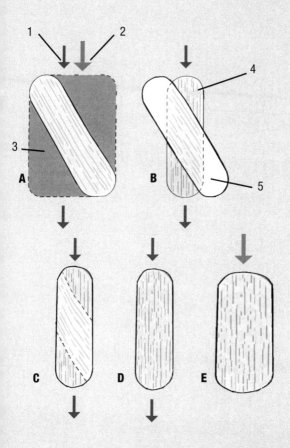

Bone Remodelling

Bone remodelling occurs in discrete areas all over the skeleton. The process is also part of the process of # repair but is an essential part of normal bone metabolism. Osteons are constantly being renewed with changing forces – age, calcium metabolism & other factors. Interference in this process may lead to pathological fractures – mineralization of other Ts & other pathology (eg OP).

RANKL – a cytokine – stimulates the process to begin, by activating the osteoclasts. It may come from the resident OCs, circulating mΦ or from the mesenchyme.

Schema of cellular processes

A Quinesence – resting bone

B Resorption – osteoclasts activated – dissolving bone matrix (~10days)

C Reversal – mΦ present in the area

D Formation – OBs recruited to form new osteoid – calcified bone matrix

E Remodelling – OCs move in remodel the bone to form laminae and new osteons

The process then returns to Quinesence

1 osteocytes = OCs

2 lining (cells of the endosteum)

3 osteoclasts = giant cells

4 osteoclasts = giant cells = GC

5 haemopoietic stem cell

6 monocyte = MNC

7 macrophage = mΦ

8 mesenchymal stem cell (CT cell)

9 osteoblast progenitor cell (OG) – prior to activation

10 osteoblasts = OBs

11 osteoid – new bone T

12 mineralized compact bone matrix

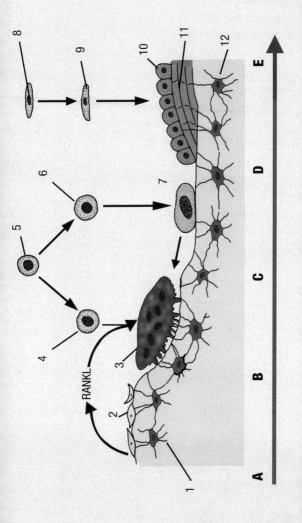

BONES in situ – Anterior

1 Frontalis – *forehead*

2 Zygoma

3 Maxilla – *upper jaw*

4 Mandible – *lower jaw*

5 Clavicle – *collar bone*

6 Humerus – *arm*

7 Manubrium

8 Sternum   – *breast bone*

9 Xiphoid process

10 Temporalis

11 Vertebrae – cervical (7) – *neck*

12 *shoulder joint*

14 *elbow joint*

15 Radius

16 Ulna   – *forearm*

17 Carpal bones – *wrist bones* (8 each hand)

18 Vertebrae – lumbar (5) – *lower back*

19 Metacarpal bones – *hand bones*

20 Phalanges – *fingers*

21 *wrist joint*

22 Femur – *thigh bone*

23 Patella – *kneecap*

24 Fibula

25 Tibia – *shin*   – *lower leg*

26 *ankle joint*

27 Phalanges – *toes*

28 Metatarsal – *forefoot bones*

29 *knee joint*

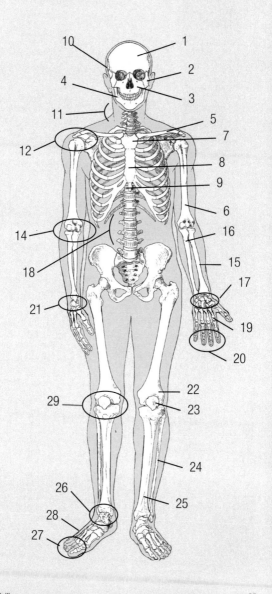

BONES in situ – Posterior

1   Parietal bone
2   Occipitalis
3   Vertebrae – cervical (7)   *neck*
4   Vertebrae – thoracic (12) – *upper back*
5   Vertebrae – lumbar (5) – *lower back*
6   Sacrum
7   Carpal bones – *wrist bones*
8   Pollux – *thumb*
9   Metacarpals – *hand bones*
10 Phalanges – *fingers*
11 Calcaneus – *heel*
12 *knee joint*
13 Ischium – part of the hip bone – "*sitting bone*"
14 *hip joint*
15 Ileum – part of the hip bone
16 12th rib – (24 ribs in total – 12 each side)
17 Humerus – *arm bone*
18 Scapula – *shoulder bone – medial edge – shoulder blade*

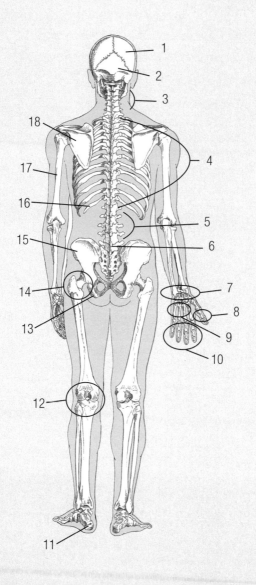

Articular cartilage structure
Hyaline cartilage

Micro cellular structure / collagen fibre orientation

Zones

I   tangential collagen fibres – i.e. along the surface

II   oblique collagen fibres – transition to the vertical collagen fibres down the length of the cartilage

I + II = hydrated zones water flows in & out of these zones – depending upon the pressure joint*

III vertical collagen fibres in cartilage

IV   calcified cartilage

V   subchondral bone

Histology

1   lamina splendens

2   chondrocyte in lacuna

3   ground substance (GS)

4   bone edge

5   end plate

6   trabecular bone

7   BM

8   collagen fibres

* it is to be noted that height is lost in the day and restored in the evening, particularly in the VC, due to water going in and out of the cartilage GS.

© A. L. Neill

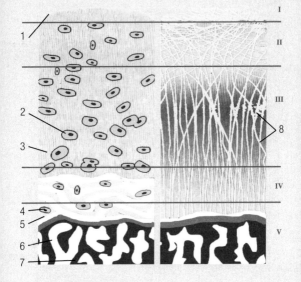

Epiphyseal plate cartilage

Histology MP

1. distal bone T of plate
2. resting cartilage cells
3. mitotic cartilage cells increasing the length of the LB
4. cells dying and matrix calcifying
5. osteoblasts depositing osseous ground substance

Schema of LB

1. EP
2. secondary ossification centre
3. cartilage
4. compact bone – shaft of the LB

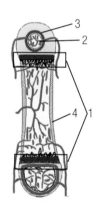

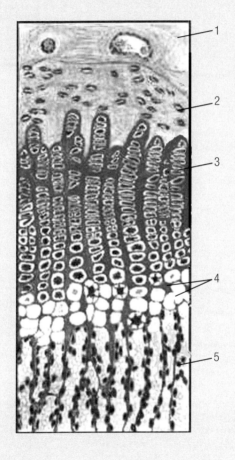

1

2

3

4

5

Classification & Summary of Joints

defn: joint = any bone something bone = B+?+B
whenever 2 or more bones meet

TYPE OF JOINT	STRUCTURE	MOVEMENT	EXAMPLES
GOMPHOSIS	BONE - FIBRES TOOTH	nil	teeth / jaw bone
SYNARTHROSES = FIBROUS JOINT	BONE - FIBRES - BONE	little / nil	
eg SUTURE (short fibrous connection b/n bones)	BONE - FIBRES - BONE	nil	joints in the Skull joints b/n flat bones
eg SYNDESMOSIS (longer fibres more cartilage)	BONE - FIBRES - BONE	little	Tibiofibula joint Radioulna joint
SYNCHONDROSIS = 1° CARTILAGENOUS JOINT (Amphiarthrosis)	BONE - HYALINE- CARTILAGE - BONE	due to the elasticity of the CARTILAGE	1st costal cartilage to the Manubrium rib cartilage Manubriosternum
SYMPHYSIS (2° cartilagenous joint)	BONE - FIBRO-CARTILAGE - BONE	little in all directions - may be influenced by HORMONES	MOST joints in axial skeleton eg b/n VERTEBRAL BODIES b/n Pubic bones
SYNOVIAL (Diarthrosis)	BONE - HYALINE CARTILAGE SYNOVIAL FLUID HYALINE CARTILAGE BONE	Full movement type depends upon the shape of the boney surfaces	MOST joints in the appendicular skeleton upper limb lower limb feet and hand joints

Synovial joint types

1	Ball & Socket	movement in many directions - common centre	hip / shoulder
2	Condyloid	movement in 2 directions	wrist / ankle
3	Hinge	one directional	elbow / knee / finger / toe
4	Pivot	movement around an axis	atlanto-axial medial joint (C1/C2)
5 (5e)	Plane (Ellipsoid)	gliding / sliding	costovertebral zygapophyseal
6	Saddle	movement in all directions except axial rotation	thumb MCP scaphoid

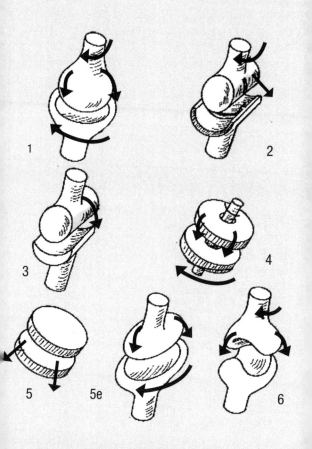

1

2

3

4

5   5e

6

Diarthrosis – Moveable Joint
Synovial joint

All bone to bone connections are joints – but those which allow for extensive movement are synovial joints. They all have several features in common, some have additional specializations as seen here.

Schema of Knee joint – lat. view

1   Femur
2   synovial membrane
3   articular surface – hyaline cartilage
4   joint space
5   cruciate ligs. = intra-articular structures – i.e. inside the joint space
6   joint capsule
7   Tibia
8   Meniscal cartilage = fibrocartilage discs = intra-articular structures
9   bursae – i = internal compartments w/n the joint space
10 Patella = knee cap
11 Quadriceps tendon
12 Quadriceps muscle

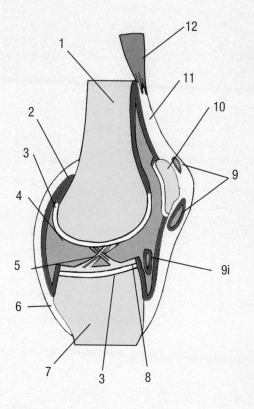

Summary of Joint movements (head to toe)
Upper body

Location	Degrees of movement	Summary – Main screening tests	
Cervical spine / Neck			
Total range ext + flex	130	limit – chin touching chest	1
hyper-Extension / Flexion	50 / 80		1
Lat flexion – R+L	45 + 45 = 90		2
Rotation	80		3
Shoulder			
Abduction	170	extended arm out to the side (90º) – then up to the head	4
Extension / Flexion	60 / 165	abducted arm (90º) extended in horizontal plane to the back / flexed to the front across the midline	5
Rotation @ 90º – external	100		6
Rotation @ 90º – internal	70		6
Rotation in extension – internal			
Elbow			
Flexion	145	fingertips to touch the shoulder	
Pronation / Supination	75 / 80	may also be referred to as "forearm movements" – combination of elbow and wrist	7

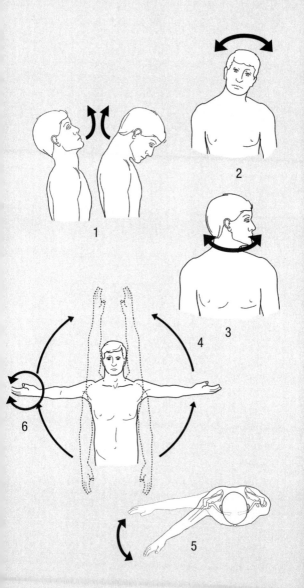

Summary of Joint movements (head to toe) Upper body continued.

Location	Degrees of movement	Summary – Main screening tests	
Wrist			
Deviation – radial/ulnar	20 / 35		8
Flexion – dorsi	75	Normal prayer position	9
Flexion – palmar	75	Inverse prayer – i.e. backs of hands together	9
Fingers			
DIP jts flexion	80		
PIP jts flexion	100		
MCP jts flexion	90	straight fingers – bent over a straight palm	
MCP jts passive hyper-extension	< 45	wrist bent backwards by examiner	
Combination		fingers to touch palm & then *tuck in*	10
Thumb			
C-MC (basal jt) palmer abduction/adduction	45	thumb to touch the little finger-tip	11
C-MC (basal jt) radial abduction/adduction	60		12
C-MC flexion	15		13
IP jt extension/flexion	20 / 80		13

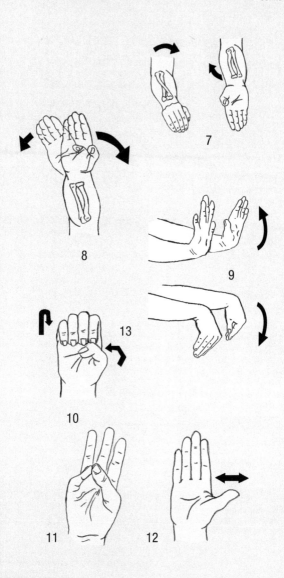

7

8

9

13

10

11   12

Summary of Joint movements – cephalo-caudally (head to toe)
Lower body

Location	Degrees of movement	Summary – Main screening tests	
Thoraco-Lumbar spine			
Flexion – lumbar / thoracic	60 / 45		14
Lat flexion – R+L	30 + 30 = 60		15
Rotation (Thoracic only) R + L	40 + 40 = 80		16
Hip			
abduction / adduction	40 / 25		17
Extension / Flexion	5–20 / 120	limited by abdomen contacting thigh if done with a flexed knee	18
Rotation @ 90° flexion – external/ internal	45		
Rotation in extension – external / internal	45 / 35		19
Knee			
Flexion	135 +	limited by heel contacting buttock	20
Ankle			
Flexion – dorsi/ plantar	15 / 55		21
Foot			
Forefoot pronation/ supination	20 / 35		
Heel eversion / inversion	10 / 20		22
The Big Toe / Great Toe			
IP jt extension / flexion	0 / 60		
MP jt extension / flexion	65/ 40		

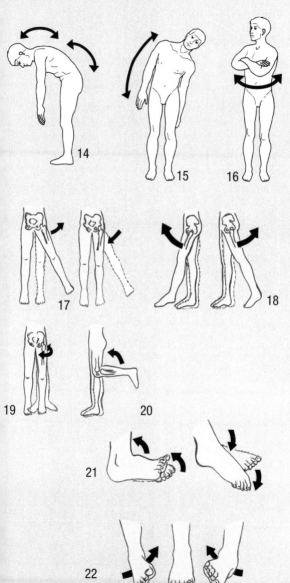

General Principles in the Orthopaedic Examination

INSPECTION

1 Shape / Posture changes

Shape and posture changes (including shortening or uneven limbs) may demonstrate – congenital abnormalities, metabolic disturbances, destructive bone / joint changes with age/time, including incorrect use of the bones as in poor posture, a form of chronic wear & tear trauma, acute trauma or a combination of all these factors.

1. poor posture
2. round shoulders
3. Dowager's hump –gen. developing from OP
4. Barrel Chest – gen. due to underlying lung disease
5. Valgus = Knock knees – gen. related to metabolic disease / or congenital
6. Vargus = Bow legs - gen. related to metabolic disease / or congenital

© A. L. Neil

2 Swelling

Swelling may be confined to a localized region of a bone or joint (as in effusions) as in: infective/inflammatory conditions, neoplastic conditions, traumatic events, or become diffuse.

These conditions may be due to a combination of any of the previously listed aetiologies

7   diffuse swelling – gen. an infection over the whole region

8   localized swelling – confined to the joint – gen. post-traumatic

9   localized swellings – present on the bones not necessarily related to the joint – gen neoplastic

10 coloured swellings – as in bruising – gen. post-traumatic or bleeding disorders

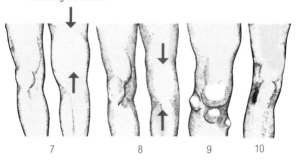

7   8   9   10

3 Wasting

Wasting may indicate disuse, from pain or disuse, 2º to N damage, which may come from neoplasia or trauma.

11   muscle wasting in upper leg – asymmetrical disuse

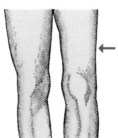

PALPATION

1 Heat in the area (which may be observed as a redness) – either localized or diffuse –both often indicate an infective inflammatory process

2 Cold particularly in distal acral regions – may indicate poor BF due to PVD or asymmetrical atherosclerosis

3 Tenderness either local or diffuse usually always indicates an inflammatory process

11 palpation for heat, maybe over a joint ± red due to ⬆ BF in the area

12 palpation for tenderness – local or diffuse with swelling may be due to pus or other inflammatory effusion

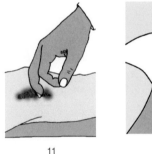

11

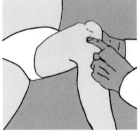

12

MOVEMENT

Nearly all orthopaedic conditions involve at least 1 jt – hence their movements need to be evaluated.

1 Test the Range of Movements (ROM) – normal

active performed by the patient - unassisted

passive performed by the examiner w/o patient input

© A. L. Neill

Generally active ROM < or = passive ROM

This needs to be recorded – ideally with the "Normal" limb – otherwise with ROM tables. "Fixed flexion deformities" – are indicative of contracting joint capsules, muscles, tendons – generally degenerative or infective processes; or of inserted masses in the region either extra-articular – indicative of neoplastic processes, or intra-articular indicative of congenital, degenerative & /or traumatic events.

2 Test the Range of Movements (ROM) – abnormal

examiner movement of the limb / jt in abnormal planes

This often indicates, structural changes – possibly due to congenital or degenerative factors

13 measuring the normal ROM of the joint

14 examination of movements in abnormal planes

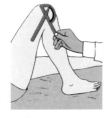

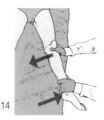

13

14

3 Detect any abnormal "clicks" or crepitus on jt movement

if this is extra-articular – it maybe soft tissues moving over the joint – clicks, if this is intra-articular – it may indicate displaced intra-articular bodies – i.e. the meniscus, or irregular joint surfaces 2° to degeneration or acute trauma

15 detection of crepitus – or a grating on movement of the jt

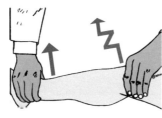

15

4 Evaluate the strength of contraction over the jt

Although not technically orthopeadic – this measurement not only determines the muscle strength but the health & strength of the underlying jt

In the LL this is particularly relevant and used to assess gait – contraction strength is determined not only by muscle strength/ wasting, but by joint pain & innervation.

on the MRC scale – strength of a contraction is scaled as

M0	no active contraction
M1	palpable contraction – but no movement
M2	weak contraction – not strong enough to counter gravity
M3	contraction can overcome gravity
M4	contraction – enables function but is not full strength
M5	full strength

Hence it is also useful to test the sensory levels in the defined region. MRC sensory scale

S0	absence of all sensory modalities
S1	deep pain sensation
S2	recovery of protective sensation, generalized – heat, pain, touch
S3	recovery of localized sensation / and recognition of objects
S4	normal sensation

16 examination of the
   sensory modalities

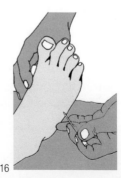

16

© A. L. Neill

Notes:

The Ankle

Anatomy – *simple hinge joint – movements in a single plane plantar / dorsiflexion + axial rotation around the Tibia up to 18° (eversion / inversion)*

Weight load – *through the Tibia & Talus*

Stability – *+++++*

A/P – *curved tibial bony prominences & ligs + weight bearing forces.*

M/L – *medial (tibial) & lateral (fibular) malleoli & ligs. includ. tibiofibular ligs. which bind the Fibula & Tibia together**

S – *superior view. When the foot dorsiflexes (df) the Talus moves backwards (see red arrows) so the wider anterior surface fits b/n the malleoli and the jt becomes more secure – the opposite is true of plantar flexion (pf)*

Fractures/tears to any of these stabilizing structures will result in failure of the ankle joint

1. weight load –load bearing forces in standing
2. Tibia – articular projections from the articular surface
   a = ant / p = post
3. Talus
4. malleolus m= medial L = lateral
5. inf. tibiofibular ligs (ant & post)
6. interosseus lig
7. Fibula
8. Calcaneus
9. lateral lig – 3 parts = External lig
10. medial lig = Deltoid lig
11. Navicular
12. Spring lig

* *More details of the structure of the ankle can be found in* **The A to Z of the bones joints & ligaments and the Back**

© A. L. Neill

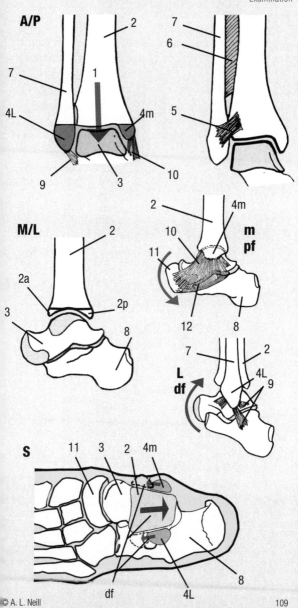

A/P

M/L

m pf

L df

S

© A. L. Neill

The Foot

Anatomy – *The foot acts as a tripod with the force direction from the Tibia going through to the triangular base - of the 1st (1) & 5th (5) MTs & the Calcaneus(2). It moves in 3 axes – X, Y & Z which use the many jts in the foot to facilitate this. Flexion & Extension in the X axis allows the foot to accommodate slopes; Abduction & adduction or turning out & in the Y axis with the feet is limited and mainly in the midtarsal jt (3) in the Y axis and Inversion & Eversion in the Z axis which allows for balance in uneven surfaces is mainly in the subtalar jt (4).*

Stability – +++++
Good with the many interlocking bone surfaces and limited range of movement along with the broad base of the foot

XYZ tripod of the foot schema

X   movements in the X plane

Y   movements in the Y axis

Z   movements in the Z axis

  1   1st metatarsal bone

  2   Calcaneus

  3   midtarsal jt

  4   subtalar jt

  5   5th metatarsal bone

** More details of the structure of the foot can be found in **The A to Z of the bones joints & ligaments and the Back***

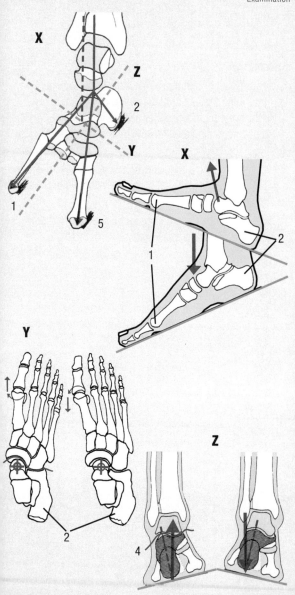

The Ankle – Radiological features

Schema A/P

A   the amount of tibiofibular overlap (1) can be used to determine the extent of diastasis, while the EP (2) should not be mistaken for a Hx of #, although the small "os fibulae" (3) can be a sign of lig &/or bone avulsion & ankle instability.

B   if the gap b/n the medial malleous & the Talus (4) > the gap of the Tibia & Talus (5) it also indicates diastasis & ankle instability

C   the presence of any defects or foreign bodies on the articular surfaces (6) indicate arthropathy – osteochondritis tali is the commonest seen in the ankle

D   note any deformaties on the bony points indicating past avulsions (7)

E   congenital deformities show up as gross deformities of the bone shape (8) – generally with a compensatory   in bone density

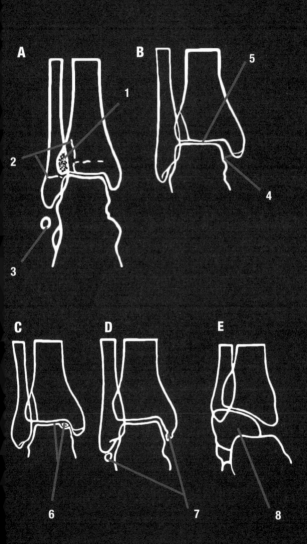

The Ankle – Radiological features

Schema – Lateral views

A   the small os trigonum (1) is a normal bony feature of the ankle not a sign of previous avulsion.

B   if the gap b/n the talar & tibial articular surfaces (2) are not circular & parallel even with careful positioning then there is subluxation & surface irregularities which may indicate arthropathy

C   anterior exostoses (3) on the Talus or Tibia are signs of stress anteriorly as in football kicking – posteriorly there may be alterations in the articular line (4) representing #s

D   generalized exostoses (5) & osteophytes (6) present around the joint indicate arthritic changes – along with narrowing and fuzziness of the joint line (7)

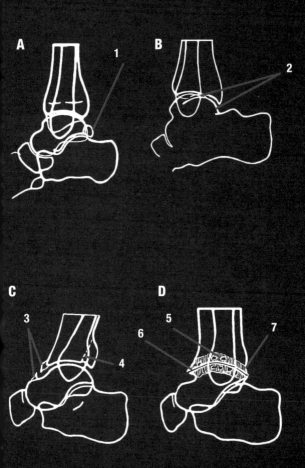

The Ankle – Inspection

Anterior

A   Scars & deformities – These may be due to previous operations – i.e. sinus drainage (1) or past fractures (2)

B   Posture deformities – plantar flexion – These may indicate shortened or ruptured tendons, partic the Achilles tendon or bone deformities generally congenital – Talipes deformity

C   Bruising & Swelling – Note if the swelling – oedema is uni or bilateral (indication of systemic disease), local or generalized

D   lateral egg-shaped lateral swelling – If this appears quickly – and is hard lateral and local – it indicates lateral lig tear

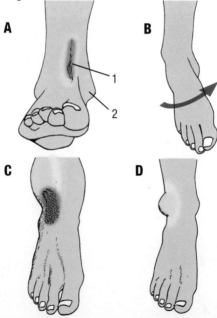

The Ankle – Inspection
Posterior

It is not possible to see a lot of the bony features from behind in the ankle because of the Archilles tendon tends to cover most of them. This is the longest (16cm) & strongest tendon in the body, essential to the functioning of the joint.

The best method to examine posterior ankle joint is to lay the patient prone on the bench & have the feet extended over the edge, comparing the normal side contour with the abnormal side.

A   upper limb NAD / lower limb shows localized swelling (1) & an exostosis (2) of the Calcaneus – (Hagland's deformity) often associated with tendinitis of the Achilles tendon.

B   in Achilles tendon rupture the tendon contour is obviously disturbed (3)

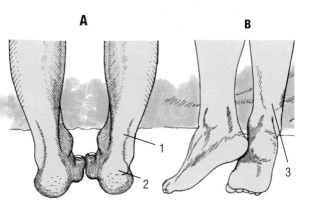

The Foot
The Big Toe – Toes Inspection

Toes show a number of deformities generally more exaggerated on the big toe but most occur in any 1 or more toes –

Hallux Rigidus *– OA of the 1st MTP of the big toe will show up with thickening of the jt (1) or a fixed flexion deformity (2) with a bunion due to poor foot posture on the sole (7). This is a common site for gout and other articulate arthropathies.*

Claw toes *if generalized indicate a primary neuromuscular problem or local intrinsic muscle problem – extended forefoot (8) with a fixed flexion of the IP jts (9)*

Corns *hard on the external surfaces (10) or soft (11) when b/n toes can occur anywhere distinguished from bunions in that they do not occur at pressure sites*

Hammer toes *– have fixed flexed PIP jts (12)*

Mallet toes *– have fixed flexed DIP jts (13)*

Curly toes *– are due to a form of fixed flexion in the IP & MTP jts (14)*

> *grade 1 – mild (14i)*
>
> *grade 2 – showing some over or under-riding (14ii)*
>
> *grade 3 – severe – concealing all of the nail from the dorsum (14iii)*

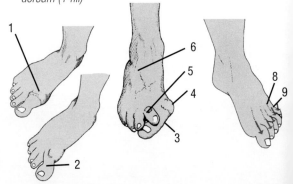

© A. L. Neil

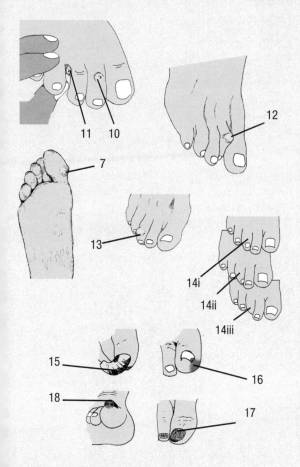

Toe nails may be painful for several reasons associated with inflammation, malformation and trauma.

deformed toenail = onychogryphosis (15)

ingrown toenail (16)

texture roughened (17)

elevated – due to subungual exostoses (18)

The Ankle – Palpation

articular surfaces

A forcible plantarflexion of the foot allows for anterior palpation of the Talus

tenderness here on examination is present in: arthritic conditions (OA)

bony exostoses (as in footballer's ankle), & osteochondritis of the Talus.

B movement of the forefoot while holding the ankle allows for the detection of crepitus present in any condition of articular damage / joint damage.

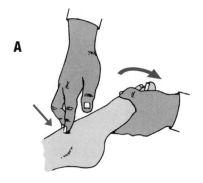

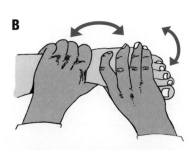

© A. L. Neill

The Ankle – Palpation

lateral ligament

A   palpation on the lateral side – tenderness here on examination is present when there is a lat. lig. tear

B   prone patient is placed with the foot over the end of the bench & the ankle pressed downwards – ⬆ movement indicates torn ant. part of the lat. lig. – note if there is dimpling of the skin around the Archilles tendon

C   stressed inversion & palpation of a gap b/n the Tibia & Talus – leg & heel bones indicates lat. lig. tears – this may be painful & require local anaesthesia & Xray for Dx

D   with the supine patient – press down on the joint to anteriorly displace the ankle – palpation of a gap b/n the Tibia & Talus – leg & heel bones indicates ant. part of the lat. lig. is torn – this may be painful & require local anaesthesia & Xray for Dx

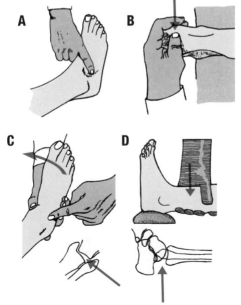

The Ankle – Palpation

posterior

Pain on the back of the ankle / leg maybe due to bone &/or tendon pain – tendinopathy

A locate the site of maximal pain by moving up the back of the ankle, gently squeezing the tendon – noting any heat or fusiform swelling. Tendon pain typically occurs 3-5cm proximal to the insertion (bone pain is typically lower and muscle pain higher).

B resisted plantarflexion will demonstrate any gap in the tendon & change its site with the movement – if the site does not change with the movement then the pain is located in the bone.

C pinching the posterior muscles will move the foot into plantarflexion if the tendon is intact, if the Achilles tendon is ruptured, it will not.

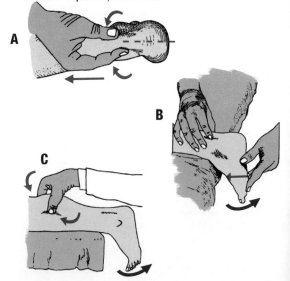

© A. L. Neill

The Ankle – Palpation

tibiofibular ligaments (ant. & post.)

A   tenderness on examination just above the ankle line anteriorly & posteriorly – indicates a tear in the inf. tibiofibular ligs

B   dorsiflexion of the foot moves the Fibula posteriorly – tenderness indicates tears in the inf. tibiofibular ligs

C   lateral displacement of the ankle – indicates tibiofibular lig tear with eversion there may be medial lig &/or Fibula involvement

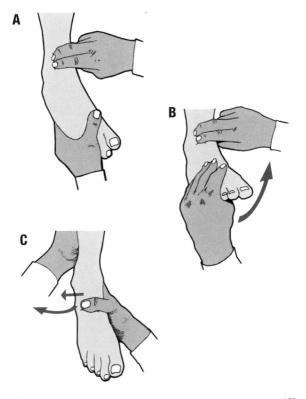

The Ankle – Palpation

tenosynovitis

The basis of examination for this condition is to find and "milk" the major tendon pathways – and place them under stress to see if this causes irritation

Medial

A examination of the major flexor tendons milking for excess synovial fluid (1)

B examine the ankle with eversion & plantarflexion for tibialis posterior (2)

C palpate along the length of the flexors noting any thickening or heat

Medial & Lateral

D examine behind both malleoli while moving the forefoot and fixing the ankle for crepitus – also auscultate

Lateral

E examine the peroneal tendons for tenderness and excess fluid – with eversion note if the tendon displaces – "snapping peroneal tendons" (3)

F plantarflexed & everted feel for tenderness along the peroneal tendons (4)

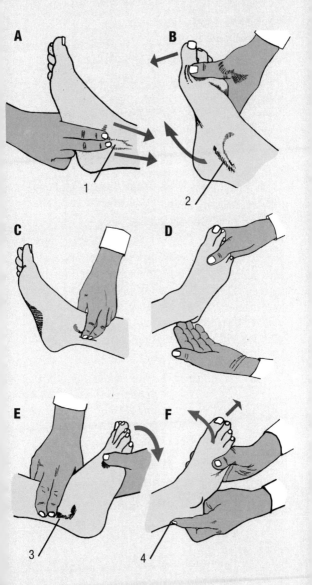

The Tender Foot
Palpation & Posture

The foot can be tender for a number of reasons.

A Tenderness in the heel is present around the Achilles' tendon (1) – particularly in children (Sever's disease) and slightly below it in adolescents (Calcaneal exostoses, bursitis) (2), and on the sole near the heel in adults (plantar fasciitis, inferior exostoses) (3).

B This in part may be due to the poor posture of the foot / heel which may be valgus (4) or varus (5) associated with pes planus and pes cavus respectively. These should correct when going up on the toes – due to muscle realignment unless there is jt dysfunction generally arthritis.

C Tenderness in the forefoot is generally due to plantar neuroma. Compressing the MTs of the forefoot will elicit pain and parasthesia if positive (Mulder's sign) (6). Further location can be made if the foot is also compressed from above & below as the examiner moves from the front to the back of the foot (7) feeling for the click – or the patient to indicate maximal tenderness.

D Tarsal tunnel syndrome is similar to carpal tunnel syndrome in that a stressed plantar surface will cause pain. To do this dorsiflex (8) & evert the foot (9) and toes. If positive this will cause pain after about 60s, particularly if the posterior tibial N, at the back of the lateral malleous, is tender (10).

Note the 1st MTP jt is very tender in Hallux rigidis, Gout and other arthroses – see the toes.

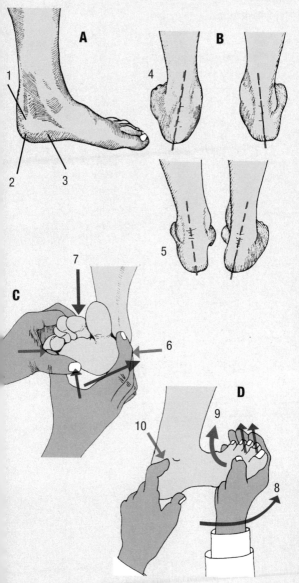

The Ankle – Movements

A before measuring the ankle movements – mobilize the joint by grabbing the heel & moving it passively – ensuring the mid & forefoot do not move

B dorsiflexion is measured actively & passively with a goniometer – NAD = 15º

   if restricted, flex the knee & note if the ROM   hence the Achilles tendon is shortened – if there is no difference it is not tendon based – but an arthropathy e.g. OA RA

C plantarflexion is measured actively & passively with a goniometer – compare if possible with the normal side NAD = 55º

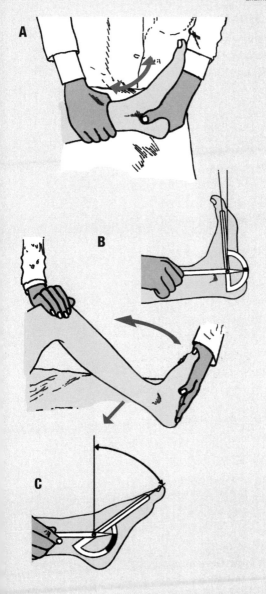

The Elbow

Anatomy *– hinge joint due to the close bony fit of the Ulna (1) and trochlea (2) (of the Humerus). In full extension the olecranon process (1p) fits snugly into the olecranon fossa (1f). In full flexion the coronoid process (1c) fits into its fossa (2l).*

Stability *– +++++ further reinforced by strong collateral ligs (4). flexion = 145° rotation = 80°*

Radio-ulnar joint *– annular lig (5a) + weaker long connecting interosseous lig (5i) pronation/supination rotate through the radial head (3) movement range extension*

Schema *E = extension (straight arm)*
F = flexion (bent arm)
P/S = pronation/supination (palms down / palms up)
L / T = ligaments & tendons
M – medial / L – lateral

1   trochlea of the Humerus

   1c   coronoid process

   1f   olecranon fossa

   1p   olecranon process

2   olecranon of the Ulna

   2f   coronoid fossa

3   head of the Radius

4   collateral ligs

5   supportive ligs

   5i   interosseus

   5a   annular

6   biceps tendon (flexion)

7   brachialis tendon (flexion)

8   triceps tendon (extension) + gravity

** More details of the structure of the elbow can be found in **The A to Z of the bones joints & ligaments and the Back** and The A to Z of Skeletal Muscles*

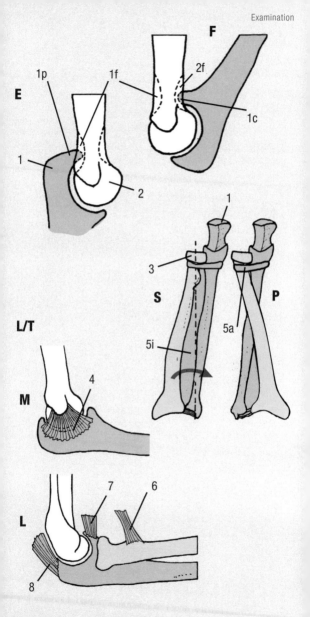

The Elbow – Radiological features
Schema normal

A   the features of the elbow jt in A P views are:
    the epicondyles lat (1L) and medial (1m), the olecranon
    and coronoid fossa (2), the capitulum (3) and radial head
    (4), the radial tuberosity (5), the capitulum (6) and the
    coronoid process of the Ulna (7).

B   the features of the elbow jt in lateral views are:
    the radial head (4), the coronoid process (7) and the
    olecranon (2).

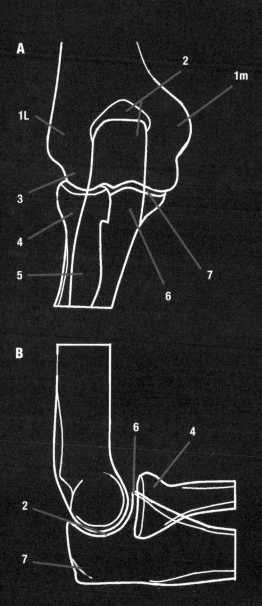

A

B

© A. L. Neill

The Elbow – Radiological features
Schema pathological features

Anterior / Posterior views

A   commonly the arthritic elbow shows osteophytes (1), joint space narrowing (2) & sclerotic jt margins (3), there may also be evidence of past #s partic with OP (4).

B   with loss of pronation/supination look for evidence of old #s & dislocations of the radial head (5)

C   the capitulum may also show signs of atrophy (6) as osteochondritis dissecans

Lateral views

D   with loss of flexion as in OA there may also be changes in the muscles / tendons as in myositis ossifcans (7)

E   loss of flexion may also be the result of previous #s which have not healed well & show bone loss (8) with poor remodelling

F   OA changes include loose bodies (9) & osteophytes (1)

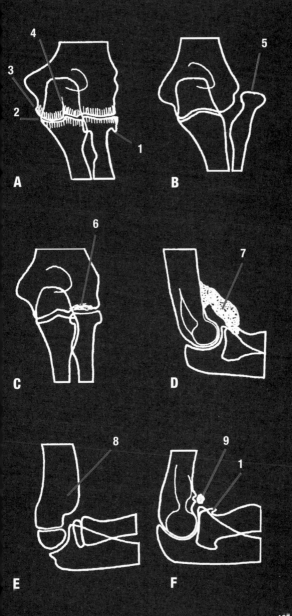

The Elbow – Inspection

1st inspection

A The generalized swollen elbow jt (1) along with muscle wasting (2) indicates an infective or arthritic condition particularly if held in the semi-flexed position – as this is the position which minimizes pain.

B Effusions begin in the hollow of the olecranon of the flexed elbow (3) and the radiohumeral jt (4) and may be squeezed b/n these 2 sites.

C Localized swellings around the olecranon – olecranon bursitis (5) or along the Ulna – rheumatoid nodules (6) also indicate pathology of the joint.

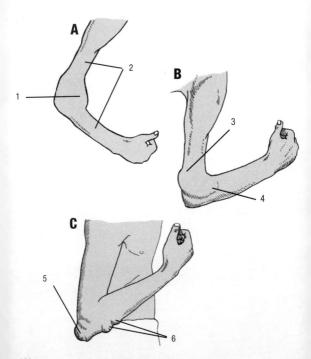

© A. L. Neill

The Elbow – Inspection

Carrying angle

A Compare the carrying angle in the standing patient to see if there are any diffierences, the commonest cause of which is previous #s.

B Cubitus valgus (1) increases the angle – cubitus varus (2) = gunshot deformity decreases the carrying angle. Variations indicate previous #s or joint laxity.

C To determine the normal angle – use the goniometer on the extended elbow.

Normal values – ♂ male 11° (2-26)
                – ♀ female 13° (3-22)

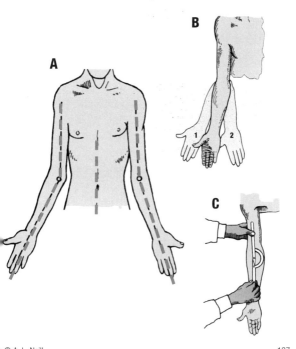

The Elbow – Palpation

A   Flexing the elbow – it is possible to locate the
    epicondyles (1) medial (1m) and lateral (1L) and the
    olecranon (2), which should form an equilateral triangle
    – unless there has been some previous injury – #s.
    Compare the carrying angle in the standing patient to
    see if there are any differences, the commonest cause
    of which is previous #s.

B   once located palpate the epicondyles – tenderness on
    the lateral indicates – tennis elbow and medial – golfer's
    elbow, i.e. tendinitis of the local ligs. Palpation of the
    olecranon indicates local bursitis or #.

C   pressing the thumb into the gap b/n the radial head and
    the Humerus – rotate the forearm (supinate / pronate)
    feeling for crepitus and/or tenderness – indicative of OA,
    injuries to the radial head or osteochondritis dissecans

D   anchoring the elbow at 30° flexion and pushing
    from side to side assesses elbow instability. If a gap
    appears on the medial side b/n the radial head and the
    Humerus (3) – valgus instability, increased laxity in the
    other direction – the less common varus instability –
    indicating lig. laxity and looseness.

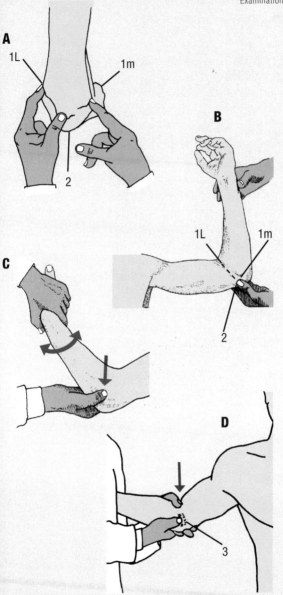

© A. L. Neill

The Elbow – Palpation 2

A flexing the elbow – it is possible to locate abnormal thickenings & masses (and loose bodies) by palpating the Jt anteriorly near the biceps tendon – as in myositis ossificans.

B suspected golfer's elbow – tendinitis on the medial side – can be detected with a flexed supinated elbow and tenderness elicited on the medial epicondyle

C suspected tennis elbow – tendinitis on the lateral side – can be detected with a pronated extended elbow and dorsiflexed clenched fist. Pressing down on the fist – to palmar flexion will elicit tenderness on the lateral epicondyles in tennis elbow (Thomson's test) – alternatively asking the patient with an extended elbow to lift a minor weight e.g. a chair will also cause pain on the lateral epicondyles – with tennis elbow.

D to examine the ulnar N it is necessary to palpate along the back of the flexed forearm, rubbing it against the Humerus. It can be seen in thin patients. Any tenderness requires a fuller neurological examination (see more details in *The A to Z of Peripheral Nerves*)

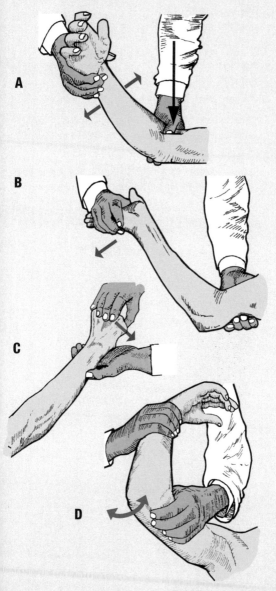

A

B

C

D

The Elbow – Movements

A   for flexion and extension ask the patient to close (1) and open their elbow jts – e.g. as in the carrying angle passively and then measure this with the goniometer for the jt ROM – compare each side for asymmetry.

B   hyperextension can be illicted after extension – with lax ligaments whereas extension is restricted in arthritic conditions

C   test pronation by fixing the elbow to the side and then turning the forearm inwards (actively and passively)

D   test supination by fixing the elbow to the side and then turning the forearm outwards (actively and passively)

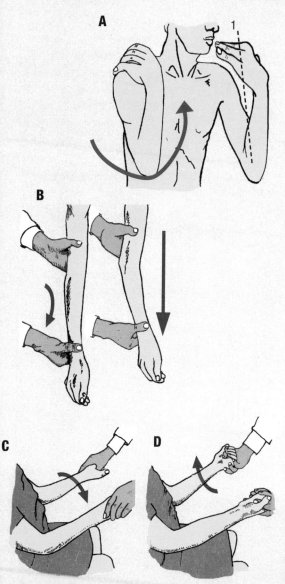

The Hand

Anatomy *– multiple joints & movements – metacarpal (hand) & phalangeal (finger) – mainly planar. The jts are covered in synovial sheaths which house the long tendons of muscles which lie primarily in the forearm to allow for fine movements unencumbered by muscle mass. W/in the hand spaces are present so that on flexion a space can develop in the hand for better function.*

The wrist is also associated and it is only an arbitrary separation of the hand & wrist in that many complaints will involve both.

Stability *– +++++ The whole hand/finger structure is a well coordinated bony group made up of very stable jts reinforced with strong ligaments, tendons & their sheaths.*

Fractures/tears to any of these stabilizing structures will result in failure of the hand's total functioning capacity.

1   distal phalange
2   interphalangeal jts (IP) - finger jts
3   metacarpophalangeal jts (MCP) – hand-finger jts
4   thenar space
5   radial bursa – synovial sheath for the thumb
6   ulnar-radial bursal communication
7   pollux tendons
8   ulnar bursa
9   midpalmar space
10 synovial sheaths (AKA tendon sheaths) of the digital tendons – fingers – note they are continuous
11 tendons – enclosed in the sheaths from forearm muscles

* *More details of the structure of the hand can be found in **The A to Z of the bones joints & ligaments and the Back***

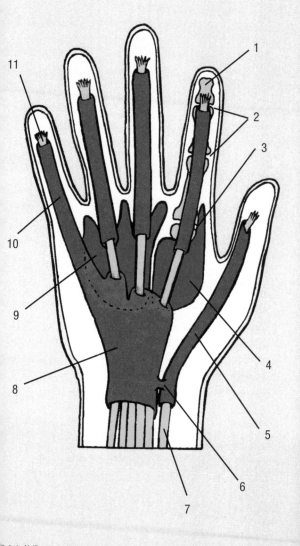

The Hand – Inspection
flexion deformities

Flexion deformities are common in the hand / fingers. They appear in various digits & to various degrees of severity & are generally due to contraction in the tendons, their sheaths &/or the fascia of the hand. If severe enough they will alter the jt(s) they cross to such an extent that full extension cannot be restored.

As with most muscle groups, the flexors are stronger than the extensors & so these deformities can also be the result of muscle imbalance, which could be of neural or vascular origin

A   flexion deformity at the MCP jt w/o extension is due to rupture of the extensor tendons – occurs at middle or ring fingers most commonly

B   flexion deformity at the PIP jt with difficult & only partial extension possible – a trigger finger – is due to tendon rupture & assoc with thickenings at the MCP jt

C   fixed flexion of the little finger of the DIP is generally congenital

D   flexion deformity assoc with hypothenar wasting (ht) is generally neural in origin & it needs to be determined if it is a local N problem or generalized neurological disorder

E   flexion of the distal IP with passive extension only is due to avulsion of the extensor tendon – 2° to trauma or RA AKA Mallet finger

F   this disorder in the thumb – Mallet thumb is due to rupture of extensor pollicus longus, 2° to trauma of the hand or wrist, RA or as a complication of a Colles' fracture

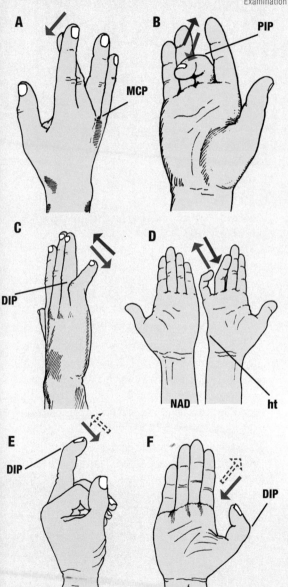

A — MCP

B — PIP

C — DIP

D — NAD — ht

E — DIP

F — DIP

The Hand – Inspection
Flexion deformities 2

Flexion deformities are common in the hand / fingers. Some are better known by their eponymous terms – e.g. Dupuytren's contracture (B), which may affect all fingers and occasionally the thumb. The palmar tendons develop nodular thickenings and contractures throughout the length of the tendon. They progress slowly compromising function & causing pain. They are often familial and return after treatment. All joints along the tendon line may be affected.

Long standing vascular compromise including PVD also causes muscle wasting & tendon contractures. This may also occur after immobilization as in #s – and present with a combination of wrist flexion and finger extension due to the tendon shortening.

A   Dupuytren's contracture – with tendon thickening (1).

B   tendon contractures may appear along the whole tendon length for example in finger (2) as well as the palm (1)

C   in Volkmann's ischaemic contracture there is clawing of the hand & fingers (3) & even the wrist (4). In the "praying position it is possible to see the gap b/n the hands (5) as the fingers cannot be fully extended. Causes include DM, PVD & brachial artery compromise.

D   wasting of the small hand muscles along with the tendon contractures lead to the classic extended finger (6) flexed hand posture (7).

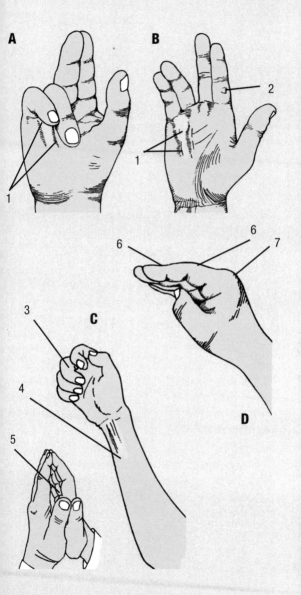

The Hand & Fingers – Infections

Infections of the hands & fingers may affect the bones tendons & jts and so are potentially dangerous to the functioning of the hand.

Fingers

A   paronychia – infection of the skin along the side of the nail (1) – is the commonest infection of the fingers, the resulting swelling causes pain due to ↑ nail plate pressure (2).

B   apical infections put pressure on the distal phalanx (3).

C   subungal exostoses (4) are DD of paronychia.

D   pulp infections (5) have the potential to destroy the bone in the distal phalanx (6).

E   tendon infections cause fusiform swelling & flexion of the affected finger (7) which resists straightening & is extremely painful. Tendon rupture may result.

Hands

F   infections of the midpalmar space or thenar eminences will cause gross swelling all over the hand – back (8) & front with greater swelling on the radial side (9) and possibly compromise the tendons crossing & MC bones. Piercing injuries are generally the cause and so look for a piercing trauma of the hand.

G   similarly wounds in the web area (10) will also cause gross swelling – this is because the anatomy of the hand / wrist (see wrist anatomy) is designed to create space for better functioning partic with grips, and is not compartmentalized.

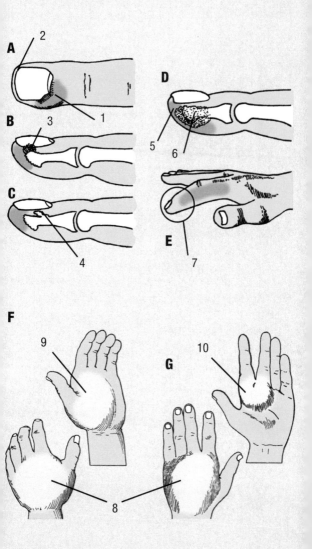

A

2

1

B

3

C

4

D

5

6

E

7

F

9

8

G

10

8

The Hand Shape – Inspection

A Achondroplasia – AKA dwarfism – all LBs are shortened & that includes phalanges - finger bones (1), which in this hand appear shorter while the carpals   wrist bones (2) are the same. DD acromegaly – where the whole hand is large & coarse; myxoedema – where the hand is fat & podgy with dry skin.

B Single or multiple fusiform swellings (3) often indicate local manifestations of disease (RA or OA) or local trauma (rupture of the collateral ligs.). DD psoriatic arthritis (mainly on the DIP) gout, sarcoidosis, syphilis or TB.

C Marfan's syndrome shows an hypertrophy of the PIP jts, (4) while the rest of the hand is in proportion. DD giantism – where all the LBs are elongated, hyperparathyroidism – where the DIPs are shortened rather than the PIPs are elongated, Down's syndrome where the little finger is incurved but not shortened giving the hand a longer look.

D Single digit hypertrophy (5) is indicative of Paget's disease, local AV fistula or neurofibromatosis.

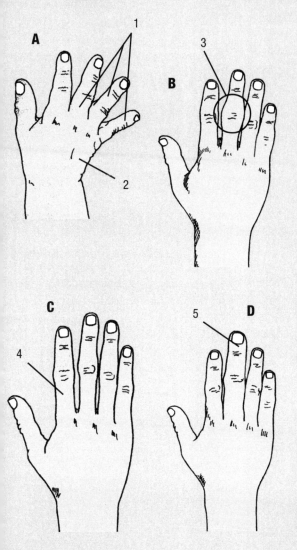

The Hand Shape – Inspection 2

Many changes occur in the hand shape due to progressive presentation of chronic diseases particularly OA & RA which target the jts in the extreme rendering them uscless.

A "Swan neck deformity" most commonly seen in the fingers of patient's with RA – DIP is flexed (1) & the PIP is hyperextended (2). Spontaneous rupture of the synovial sheaths is seen in this disease as well as tightening of the Interossei – & other intrinsic hand muscles.

B "Z deformity" is the equivalent process as above in the thumb (3).

C "Ulnar deviation" due to contraction of the ligs and tendons in the hand is progressive if untreated & may become so severe as to cause dislocation of the MCP jts (4). It is almost pathomnemonic of RA.

D Contributing & in association with to the above deviation may be specific swellings in DIPs AKA Heberden's nodes (5) associated with OA partic if it is coexisting with RA. Swellings of the PIPs AKA Bouchard's nodes (6) are a similar phenomenon.

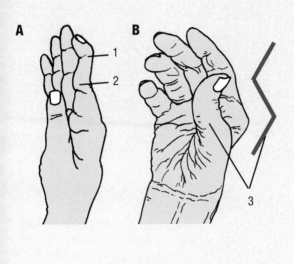

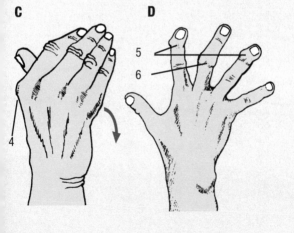

The Hand Shape – Inspection
Swellings & Nodules

Isolated swellings in the hand are most commonly due to RA but tumours which are rare in the hand may be present and need to be considered – the commonest of these is the Enchondroma.

A   Isolated swellings of the hand (1) & fingers (2), need to be investigated. If spongy with an Hx of pain the are most likely RA nodules.

B   Radiology will reveal the type of swelling – if lucent (see Pathology lucent bone images) in the hand they may be an isolated Enchondroma (3).

C   Enchondromas – benign but invasive cartilage tumours are painless and may present as a pathological #(s). If multiple (4) – multiple enchondromatosis – there is often a family Hx of their occurrence, and if treated they may reappear – AKA Ollier's disease.

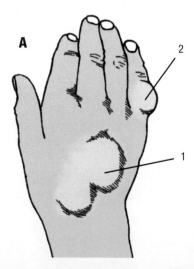

© A. L. Neill

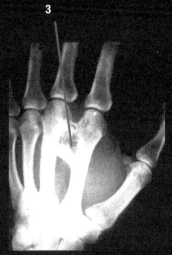

B

3

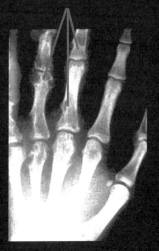

C

4

The Wrist – Palpation

Pain & swelling in the wrist is commonly the result of compressed structures passing through the flexor retinaculum – tunnel syndromes, or from the sequelae of Colles' fracture which frequently do not heal well – the resulting ulnar prominence further restricting movement & function.

A   with thumb & index finger press firmly onto the median N & time the time it takes to cause parasthesia &/or pain (16sec average with Carpal tunnel syndrome).

B   press onto the hypothenar eminence & ulnar N capsule – to determine if there is Ulnar tunnel syndrome – note if the little finger flexes or tingles in response.

C   grasp the wrist along the joint line of the Radius & Carpal bones, moving it around for tenderness & to test for jt laxity – which causes wrist weakness & generalized hand & wrist pain. Note if there is an ulnar prominence – resulting from a previous Colles' fracture.

D   palpate the anatomical snuff box to determine if there is a fracture of the Scaphoid

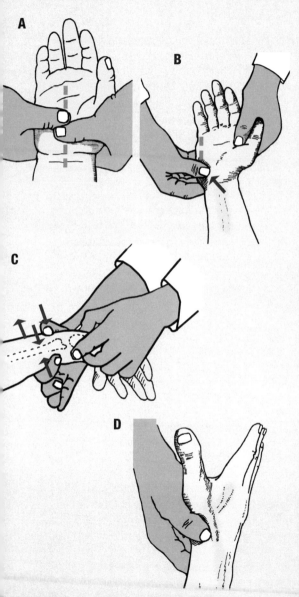

The Hip

Pattern of pathological presentation – *the hip is the major weight bearing joint in the body. The synovial joint generally discussed is the ball & socket b/n the femoral head & the hip acetabulum. From infancy to old age the pathology may be mapped chronologically i.e. the common pathologies peak at various decades and so can be predicted.*

CHD – congenital displacement of the hip AKA developmental displacement of the hip. Defn – the femoral head is not placed in the acetabulum but sits higher or more anteriorly. It presents at birth & in infancy, particularly in breech births. It is familial. It may present later in the infant or child. If missed patients may present as adults (ACHD) because of 20 OA changes, pain & loss of function. > ♂ X4

PD – Perthes' disease – avascular necrosis of the head of the femur Defn – deterioration the BS to the head of the Femur. It results in a number of malformations of this head & jt. ♂ > ♀ X5

TS – transient synovitis – If of the synovium of the hip jt Causes are: ideopathic, infective & post-traumatic.

TB – tuberculosis of the hip – rare

RA – Rheumatoid arthritis – This may affect both hips & knees in the older patient & coexist with OA. It is more severe in the younger patient AKA Still's disease (SD).

IA – infective arthritis AKA acute pyogenic arthritis of the hip – This rare disease is generally due to blood borne Staphlococcus which lodges in the hip jt space causing severe pain & affecting all movements

SFE – slipped femoral epiphysis Defn – the dislocation & movement of the head downwards from the Femur causing coxa vara ♂ > ♀ X5

AS – Ankylosing Spondylitis – rare but along with Reiter's syndrome may present first in the hip with pain & LOF

LBP – low back pain – generally due to prolapsed disc

OA – osteoarthritis – If primary OA this presents later than if associated with other diseases where the jt has had additional stresses for years

– fractures – generally due to activity in normal bone these present earlier than the pathological #s of OP & other pathologies.

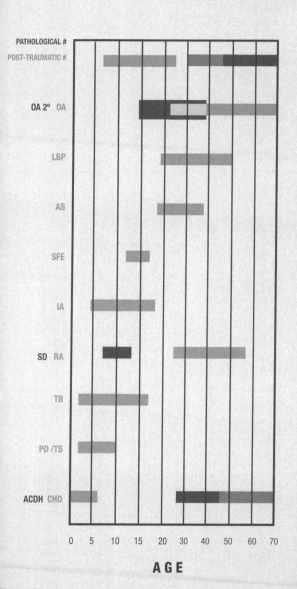

PATHOLOGICAL #
POST-TRAUMATIC #

OA 2° OA

LBP

AS

SFE

IA

SD RA

TB

PD /TS

ACDH CHD

0   5   10   15   20   30   40   50   60   70

A G E

The Hip – radiology schema

Anatomy – ball & socket joint – extensive ROM.

Weight load a lot of the weight is transferred through the neck of the Femur.

Stability – +++++ close articulating surfaces, supportive outer ligs

Radiology views of hip – NAD

A   A / P extension – bilateral

B   L view articulating surfaces – anterior

C   A / P from a superior aspect – concentrating on 1 jt

1   acetabulum

2   femoral head

3   femoral neck

4   greater trochanter

5   lesser trochanter

6   ischial tuberosity

7   femoral shaft

8   pelvic opening

9   ileum

10 pubic bone medial facet

11 obturator foramen

12 Sacrum

*   More details of the structure of thehip can be found in **The A to Z of the bones joints & ligaments and the Back**

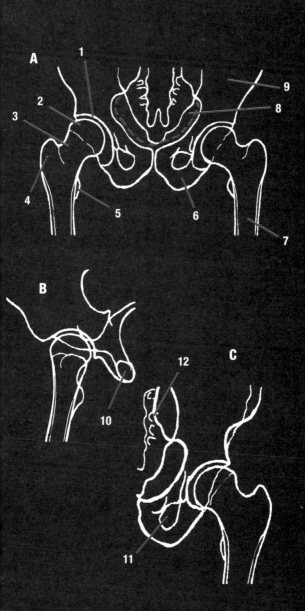

The Hip – radiology schema

Radiology views of the hip – Pathological features

In the radiological views of the hip compare with the "normal" side & note changes in :

A　⬆ jt spce (1) - as in Perthe's disease, synovitis, In present in the younger patients

B　⬇ jt space (2) – as in Ins & OA – present in the older patient

Looking specifically at the femoral head note textural changes:

C　⬇ density (3) as in OP, RA & In

Note the outline of the head in the socket

D　ragged (4) in; OP & localized avascular necrosis

Note if the head is even present or grossly deformed as in

E　Perthe's disease (5) or slipped femoral heads

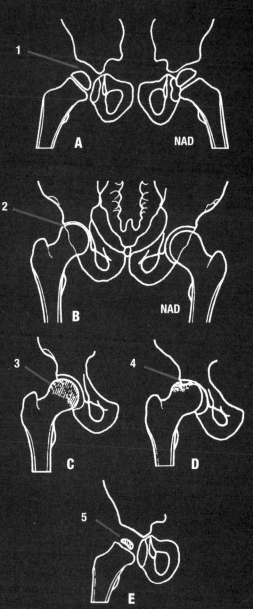

The Hip & Femur

There are specific features of the hip jt which indicate the angulation & femur placement & these can be determined from radiographs

Neck-shaft angle

Draw a line along femur shaft & along the centre of the head = neck-shaft angle (1).

The angle determines the angle of the Femur, the knee alignment and the tilt of the hip. It is vital for the functioning of the entire lower limb.

♀ 128° / ♂ 127° which along with the fact most males are taller than females – means that there is a significant ♠ angulation in the hips & knees of ♀ > ♂.

A   Coxa Vara

B   NAD – normal angle of Femur

C   Coxa Valga

Shenton's line

Normally a smooth curve will flow from the superior pubic ramus (2) to the neck of the Femur. If there is a dislocation, fracture or subluxation this line will be distorted (3).

D   Shenton's line normal

E   distorted

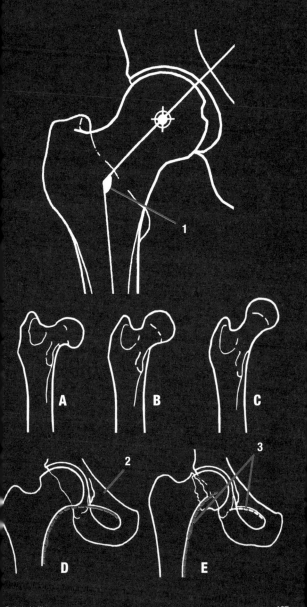

© A. L. Neill

The Hip – Shortening
Inspection

The hip jts are often asymmetrical – one "leg" appearing shorter than another.

On inspection there are several clues to this occurrence.

A   The patient often a child is seen to compensate – by either lifting the foot from the floor on the shorter abnormal leg (1) – or bending the longer normal leg (2).

B   Posteriorly the spine may twist – scoliosis (3) tilting the pelvis & so making the legs appear to have different lengths – apparent leg shortening – as opposed to true leg.

C   To determine if it is a pelvic muscle problem or a true leg shortening – lay the patient supine on the bed & level the ASIS on each side (4) to remove any effect of pelvic tilt – a true shortening will appear if the heels are not level (5).

D   There are several components to the shortening of a limb – lifting the legs to ~30° with the heels on the bed – note the level of the knee on the abnormal leg – if the knee is lower – femoral shortening (6) – if the knee is higher – tibial shortening (7).

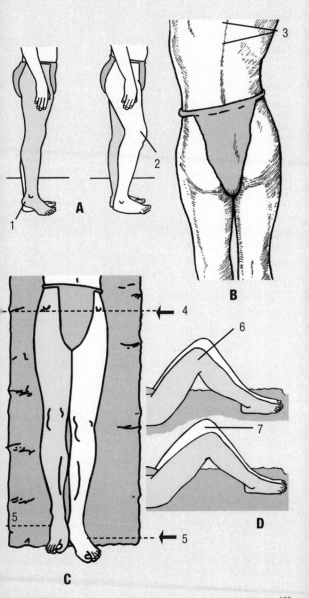

A

B

C

D

The Hip – Examination of Movements
Palpation

Movements at the hip are often a combination of the hip & the pelvis moving in concert, so to examine the "hip" movements in isolation it is important to stabilize the pelvis – generally by fixing the ASIS.

Combining movements with 2 legs at once allows for comparison & is another way to isolate the hip movements from the pelvic movements. Similarly flexing the knee to 90°

After asking for the patient to go through the routine hip movements as much as possible while standing – it is then important to re-test these with the examiner in order to measure & compare the ROM of each hip, using the normal hip as a guide. Limitations on the normal ROM occur with dislocations, hip fusion, Ins, RA & OA.

A   Abduction – fix the normal hip by locking the leg over the bench and then abducting the hip as much as possible. NAD = 40°

B   Adduction – lift the abnormal hip over the normal hip & adduct (slight flexion should not alter the measurement) NAD = 25°

C   Extension – flex & hold the normal leg to eliminate the lumbar lordosis & stabilize the hip; examine the other side to see if the leg can remain flat on the bed if it is raised it is in fixed flexion.

D   Flexion – flex & hold the normal leg to eliminate the lumbar curve & stabilize the hip; the tested leg is then flexed NAD = 120°

E   Rotation – external, cross flexed knees & hips opening up the hip space with inverted feet – compare sides – NAD = 45°   1st limitation detected in arthritic conditions

F   Rotation – internal, hold flexed hips & knees together (closed hip space) & evert the feet – compare sides – NAD = 45°

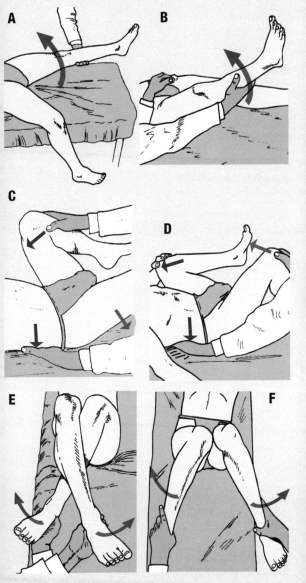

The Knee

Anatomy – 3 articulations: lateral tibiofemoral (1) medial tibiofemoral (2) & patellofemoral (3), in a common synovial sheath – or jt capsule (4), which extends into the quadriceps muscle superiorly (4s) and laterally around the sides.

Extensive number of ligaments & intra-articular structures present, a network of connecting bursae surround the joint, which allows for fluid accumulation & knee effusions to develop.

A   articulating surfaces – anterior

B   joint capsule – anterior

C   joint & bursae – medial

D   joint & burase – lateral

1   lateral tibiofemoral articulation

2   medial tibiofemoral articulation

3   patellofemoral articulation

4   joint capsule

    4d   deep patellar bursa

    4g   bursa of gastrocnemius muscle

    4i   infrapatella bursa

    4m   bursa of the semimembranous muscle

    4p   pre-patella bursa

    4s   suprapatella pouch

    4g + 4m = Baker's cyst enlarged swelling found in the popliteal fossa caused by obstruction of the flexure

5   patella ligament

6   quadriceps tendon

7   Patella = kneecap

8   Tibia

9   Fibula

10   Femur

11   gastrocnemius muscle

** More details of the structure of the knee can be found in **The A to Z of the bones joints & ligaments and the Back***

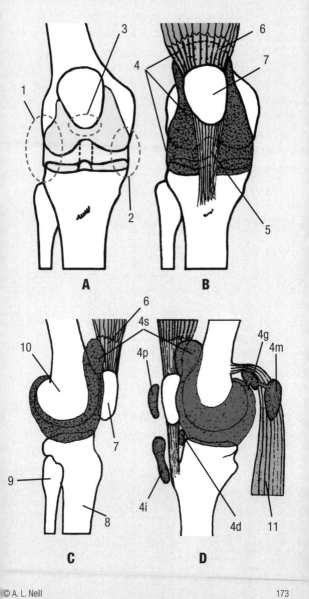

A

B

C

D

The Knee

Anatomy – cartilages (menisci) & ligaments.

The menisci help to disperse the load forces and the ligs. keep the articulating surface in place. These include the powerful collaterals (8), posterior (9) & the patella lig. anteriorly (not shown), externally & the internal cruciate ligs. (6).

A **bones & menisci – in flexion – medial**

B **bones, ligaments & menici – superior**

C **bones & menisci – in extension – medial**

D **bones & menisci – in extension – anterior**

E **bones & ligaments – in extension – lateral**

1 Femur

2 Tibia

3 Patella

4 Fibula (not part of the knee jt)

5 Meniscus – C shaped avascular fibrocartilagenous T – note the outer higher rims attached to the tibial plateau / inner concave rims remain free to move &/or compress with knee movements
5L lateral – horns attached to the tibial plateau + the Femur posteriorly
5m medial – horns attached to the tibial plateau ONLY

6 Cruciate ligaments 6a anterior – ant. tibial plateau ➡ post of the lat. femoral condyle / 6p posterior post. tibial plateau ➡ ant of the medial femoral condyle

7 meniscial lig
Going from extension ➡ flexion causes the menisci to slide anteriorly to disperse the weight of the Femur & support the bony surfaces. In the last 10º there is a medial rotation to lock the knee and this tightens the cruciate (crossing ligs). The popliteus muscle loosens this locking by lateral rotation, before flexion begins.

8 collateral ligs 8L lateral / 8m medial

9 posterior lig

* *More details of the structure of the knee can be found in **The A to Z of the bones joints & ligaments and the Back***

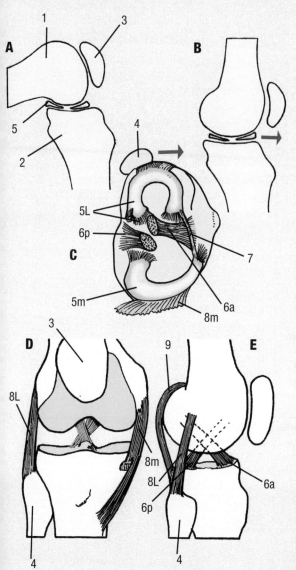

The Knee – radiology schema
Radiology views of the knee – NAD

A   *A/P extension*

B   *L view partial flexion*

A   **bones & menisci – in flexion – medial**
B   **bones, ligaments & menici – superior**
C   **bones & menisci – in extension – medial**
D   **bones & menisci – in extension – anterior**
E   **bones & ligaments – in extension – lateral**

1   Femur
    L = lateral condyle, m = medial condyle
2   Tibia
    L = lateral plateau – observe the single firm line &
    articulates with (3) 2t tibial tubercle
    m = medial plateau – double line due to the concavity
3   Fibula (articulates with 2L)

4   Patella – weaker outline in AP because of tendons
5   Fabella – normal but variable sesamoid bone of gastrocnemius
    – not a loose body

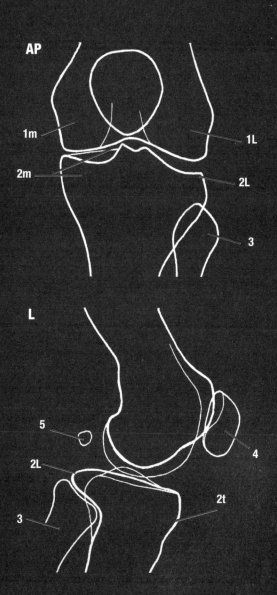

AP

1m

1L

2m

2L

3

L

5

4

2L

2t

3

© A. L. Neill

The Knee – radiology schema

Radiology views of the knee – Pathological features

A A/P extension

B L view partial flexion

C L view extension

D intercondylar tunnel view ext / flex

    De = extension

    Df = flexion

1 jt space narrowing – (indicates cartilage loss)

2 lipping (present in OA & other degen. diseases)

3 marginal sclerosis

4 cysts & lucent bodies (may indicate tumour)

5 loose bodies (OA or particulate arthritis – gout etc)

6 bipartite Patella – do not confuse with a #

7 calcified meniscus

8 marginal sclerosis

9 epiphyseal line – do not confuse with a hairline #

10 periosteal reaction – (reaction to ln or #)

11 textural changes – (indicates Paget's)

12 Patella alta – (indicating instability found in dislocations)

13 intercondylar tunnel (calcification here always path.)

© A. L. Neill

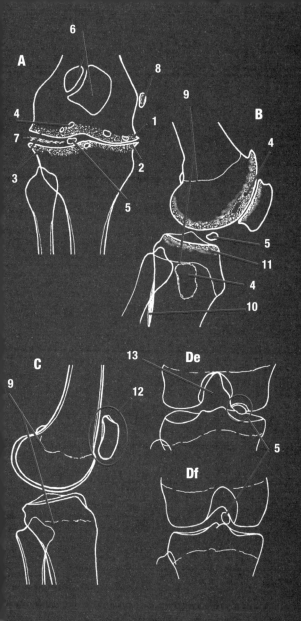

The Tibia – radiology schema
Radiology views of the Tibia – Pathological features

Pathology of the metaphysis

A   osteoclastoma

B   Brodie's abscess

C   tibial tuberosity avulsion = Osgood Schlatter disease

Pathology of the tibial shaft – shape changes

D   pseudoarthosis of the Tibia – ⬆ angulation & thinning – eventual dislocation (1)

E   Paget's disease – softening & thickening of the shaft – changed texture (2)

F   rickets – bending (3) & angulation of the ankle (4) – with weight bearing

Pathology of the tibial shaft – masses, lucent lesions

G   lytic lesions in the shaft (5) – represent neoplasia or infections

H   generalized new bone formation of the cortex – osteitis (6)

I   localized new cortical bone formation (7) – indicate reaction to stress fractures

J   circumscribed lytic lesions = unicameral bone cyst

K   with a central nidus (8) – osteoclastoma of the shaft

L   thickened cortex – indicates a healed fracture site (9)

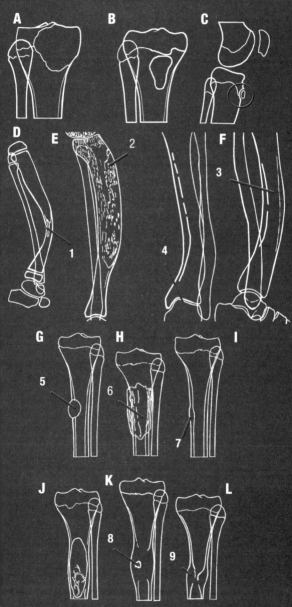

The Knee – Effusions
Inspection, palpation & examination

The knee is very susceptible to effusions – swellings. It has many bursae & spaces surrounding the jt surfaces. When the knee swells initially the hollows on the side of the knee fill – around the patella lig. (1), then the suprapatellar pouch distends (2).

To determine if the swelling above the knee is an effusion-palpate ~15cm above the knee & try to "squeeze" or empty the fluid. If it is rubbery or thickened it could be the synovial membrane (3) which has swollen in diseases such as OA & RA (G). If it is boggy & cannot be squeezed; it could be Haemarthrosis – blood in the jt space. If it is tender; it could be Pyarthrosis – pus in the jt.

Once emptied – try to push the fluid from one side to the other of the Patella while restricting the suprapatellar space (E). This will give an estimate of the extent of effusion. In fatter knees – surround the Patella with fingers & thumb and try by pushing any "fluid" present to generate a wave into the suprapatellar space (F).

A   knee lat view NAD

B   filling of the knee's lateral hollows

C   filling of the suprapatellar pouch

D   emptying the suprapatellar pouch

E   transferring fluid in the lateral hollows while restricting the suprapatellar space

F   containing the fluid in the knee – & then transferring it to the suprapatellar space

G   bogginess in the suprapatellar pouch due to swollen synovial membrane cannot be "emptied" into other spaces

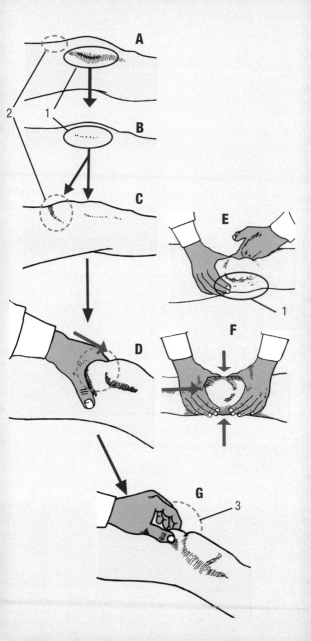

The Knee – Extensor apparatus

The extensor mechanism of the knee consists of: force through the quadriceps muscle ➡ quadriceps lig ➡ Patella ➡ patellalig ➡ tibial tubercle. Any break in this line of force results in ⬇ extension.

Any extensor weakness results in: ⬆ instability, jt trauma & effusion & PAIN.

Pain causes:

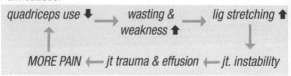

quadriceps use ⬇ → wasting & weakness ⬆ → lig stretching ⬆

MORE PAIN ⬅ jt trauma & effusion ⬅ jt. instability

Full extension is lost and then the knee cannot "lock" in full extension and tighten the knee ligs which further stretch & weaken & quadriceps further waste.

Breaks can occur at 4 places

A   rupture of quadriceps tendon

B   Patella #s

C   rupture of patella tendon

D   avulsion of the tibial tubercle

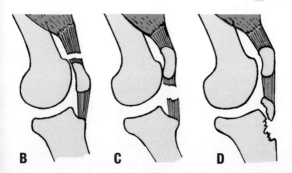

A

B   C   D

The Knee – Extensor apparatus
Palpation

If any of the components in the extensor apparatus are suspected of rupture. Palpate the extended knee in the following fashion. Commencing at the upper patella border push down until there is soft T resistance. The absence of this indicates lesion A. Moving distally – determine the site of tenderness or the presence of gaps to differentiate b/n lesions B, C & D.

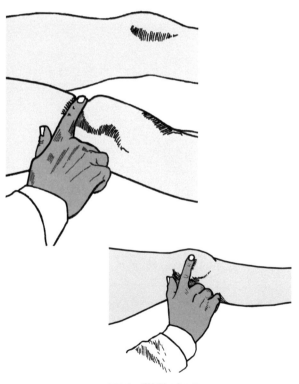

see also *Tibial tenderness*

The Knee – Meniscal failure
Inspection & examination

The menisci are fibrocartilagenous discs w/o a BS – hence injuries repair badly & occur often – particularly in sport. Generally an injury of stress with a partially flexed knee is the cause of younger injuries – footballer's knee.

Acute meniscal damage – does not bruise – but oedema on the jt line is indicative of acute or repeated damage. There are a number of dynamic tests to evaluate these injuries not discussed here. However Meniscal damage occurs in arthritic & degenerative diseases along with deterioration of the articular surfaces – also cartilage. All injuries to a meniscus can be detected with the following tests.

A screening – suspected meniscal injuries are picked up by pain along the joint line accompanied by a "springy"/bouncy resistance to full extension.

   Anteriorly with a finger on the jt line – extend the knee. Pain & clicking indicate anterior damage.

B with a fully flexed knee – place the fingers & thumb on the jt line & ask the patient to extend – any clicking coming from the jt will be detected – posterior meniscal damage can be detected this way.

C with a fully flexed knee – & palpating along the jt line place – abduct & extend the lower leg, while rotating the foot outwards. Clicks & pain will are positive indications of medial meniscal tears. (McMurray's test). A grinding is indicative of degenerative disease involving menisci &/or articular surfaces

D in the same position – adduct & internally rotate the foot to detect lateral meniscal damage &/or degenerative changes

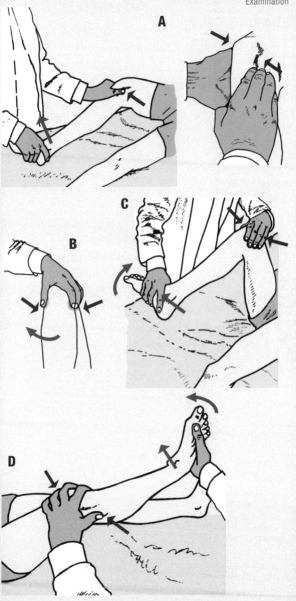

The Knee – Patella instability AKA
Patellofemoral instability

A The Patella has a lateral force (LF) when the knee extends due to the quadriceps insertion (3) & its line of contraction force – QF the site of the tibial tuberosity (4), but lateral dislocation is stopped by the femoral sulcus (1).

B Contractures in the quadriceps or ...

C an altered Q angle (2) due to a broad pelvis or knock knees – overcome this & also allow lat. displacement.*

D Hypoplasia of any of the bony components &/or repeated patella dislocations ⬆ lat. displacement

E A high sitting patella (patella alta) (5) or knee hyperextension (genu recurvatum) stops the Patella from engaging the condyles & so allow lat. displacement.

Lateral displacement leads to knee jt instability & contributes to extension mechanism breakdown.

* In knock knees an ⬆ Q angle (normally up to 6°) will predispose the patient to ant. knee pain, recurrent dislocation & chondromalacia patellae.

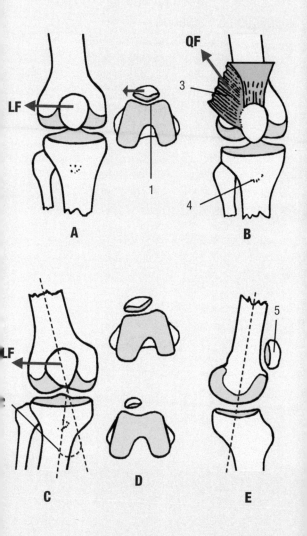

LF

QF

3

1

4

A

B

LF

5

C

D

E

The Knee – Patella Failure
Inspection & Palpation

A   examine the knees flexed over a bench – observe any asymmetry (1) which may show tibial, femur or patella deformity. Ask the patient to extend the knee from this position & note if the Patella tracks evenly. (2)

B   observe the standing patient for knock knees (Bk) = genu valgum or bowlegged (Bb) = genu varum, both of which are common in adolescent girls. Normal range of knee cap separation with legs together & Patella facing forward is < 5cm for ♂ & < 4cm for ♀.

C   examine the Patella surface all over, including the insertion sites of the tendons, the tibial tuberosity & the jt lines. Tenderness may indicate: arthritis, bipartite (split) patella, #s & faults in the extensor mechanism.

D   in order to examine the inferior surface – displace the Patella laterally then medially 2/3 of the inf. surface may be examined this way & tenderness indicates bone / surface disease.

E   relaxing the quadriceps – push the Patella around to check its mobility – then repeat while pushing the Patella hard against the femoral condyles. Pain will indicate arthritis &/or chondromalacia patellae.

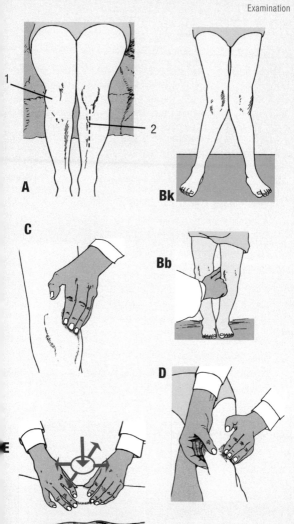

The Knee – Instability

The knee is inherently unstable & relies on the integrity of the supportive ligs – if they are torn then there is a resulting instability of this jt. There are several main types of instability. Basically a single lig tear will result in one of 4 directional instabilities – and multiple tears result in rotational instabilities.

Grade 1 tears – when the lig is stretched but not torn – showing tenderness but no laxity

Grade 2 tears – when the lig is torn

Grade 3 tears – when more than 1 lig is torn

A   Valgus instability – when the medial collateral lig is torn – so the knee may be moved laterally – forming knock knees under stress – grade 3 also involves the posterior cruciate lig.

B   Varus instability – when the lateral collateral lig is torn – so the knee may be moved medially – forming bow legs under stress – grade 3 also involves the posterior cruciate lig.

C   Anterior displacement of the Tibia – where the anterior cruciate lig is torn – so the knee moves forward – grade 3 also involves either lat &/or medial ligs.

D   Posterior displacement of the Tibia – where the posterior cruciate lig is torn – so the knee moves backward – grade 3 also involves the lat &/or med ligs.

Grade 3 tears also involve a rotational instability

anteromedial instability

anterolateral instability

posteromedial instability

posterolateral instability

Grade 4 – is when there is an associated bone avulsion

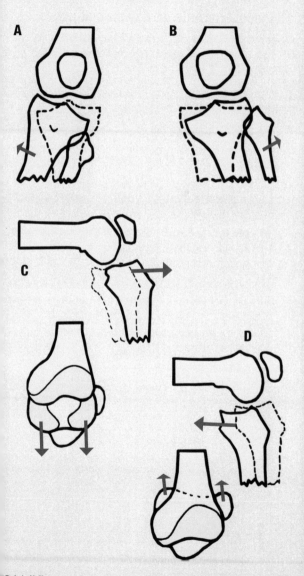

The Knee – Anterior instability
Examination - Anterior drawer test

The knee is inherently unstable & relies on the integrity of the supportive ligs – if they are torn then there is a resulting instability of this jt.

In suspected damage to the ant. cruciate ligament (AC), place the patient on the bed & flex the knee to 90°, feet facing forwards. This is later repeated with inversion & eversion of the foot if the involvement of other ligs is also suspected.

A   In the relaxed leg – pull hard on the knee with thumbs on the tibial tubercle (1). If the knee moves forward > 1.5cm – suspect medial collat. lig involvement as well – repeat with foot in 30° eversion. If the Tibia rotates as well as travelling forward suspect lat. lig involvement – repeat with 30° foot inversion.

B   There may also be damage to the post cruciate lig (PC) – if this is the case – the Tibia may have already displaced posteriorly (Bp) – giving an exaggerated or false +ve drawer test (Ba) – so it is essential to inspect the knee contour for this prior to testing.

see also Knee posterior instability

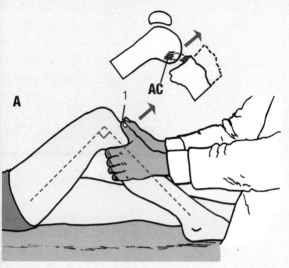

A

AC

1

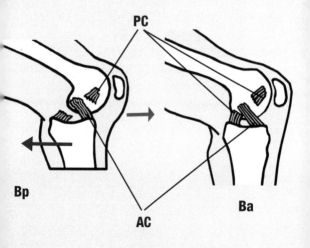

PC

Bp

Ba

AC

The Knee – Lateral instability
Varus – instability = Lateral instability – examination

The knee is inherently unstable & relies on the integrity of the supportive ligs.

A   examine the knees flexed over a bench – observe any obvious asymmetry; press on the lateral joint line particularly on the head of the Fibula; if there is tenderness but no laxity – it indicates stretching of the lig. but no tearing. Grade 1

B   if it is lax as well – place the patient on the bed & stabilizing the knee – attempt to push the knee inwards (adduction) – look for varus & an ↑ in the joint space. Grade 2

    if there is an opening of the jt space – attempt to displace the Tibia – if it is possible to push it anteriorly then this is anteriolateral instability – Grade 3

    if it is possible to displace the Tibia posteriorly then this is posterolateral instability – Grade 3.

C   note also test active dorsiflexion of the foot – to determine if the motor fibres of the common peroneal N (AKA lateral peroneal N) have been damaged.

© A. L. Neill

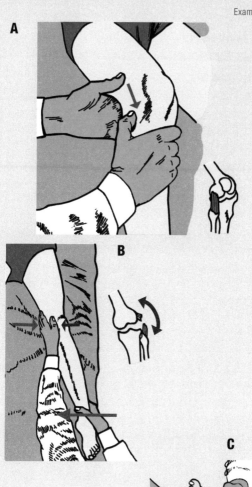

The Knee – Medial instability
Valgus – instability = Medial instability – examination

The knee is inherently unstable & relies on the integrity of the supportive ligs – if they are torn then there is a resulting instability of this jt. One of the commoner injuries is medial lig damage.

A examine the knees flexed over a bench – observe any obvious asymmetry. press on the joint line & if there is tenderness but no laxity – it indicates stretching of the lig. Grade 1

B if it is lax as well – place the patient on the bed & stabilizing the knee – attempt to push the knee outwards (abduction) – look for valgus & an ⬆ in the joint space. Grade 2

C if there is an opening of the jt space – attempt to displace the Tibia – if it is possible to push it anteriorly then this is anteriomedial instability – Grade 3

if it is possible to displace the Tibia posteriorly then this is posteromedial instability – Grade 3.

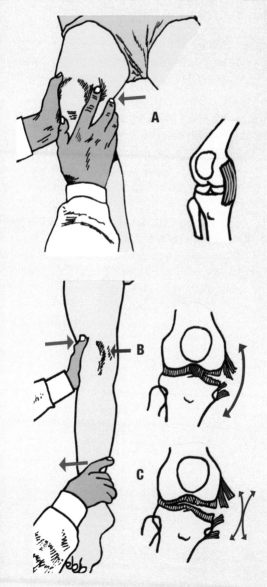

The Knee – Posterior instability
Inspection & examination

Posterior cruciate lig damage is often able to be detected with inspection alone.

A   examine the knees flexed ~ 20° over a pillow or sandbag – observe any obvious asymmetry. The deformity of the affected knee moving backwards can be quite striking (1). Grade 3

B   If the patient extends their knees the anterior movement of the Tibia will correct this deformity, if it is due to the post. lig.

C   to check further – push downwards in the same flexed position and determine if there is a resulting post. displacement – Grade 1-2. (see also anterior instability)

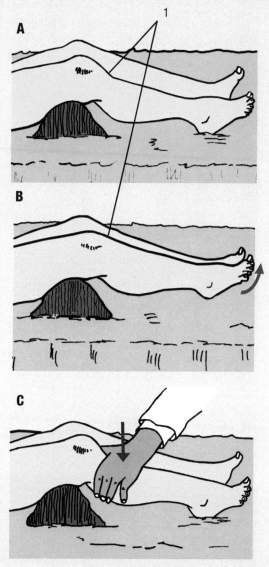

1

A

B

C

© A. L. Neill

The Tibia – Tenderness

The Tibia is very susceptible to injury & pain.

A   ant. view of the Tibia

B   post. view of the Tibia

1   tenderness over the tibial tuberosity is indicative of: Osgood-Schlatter disease (tuberosity avulsion in the adolescent), Patella tendon stress, pain of the inf. pole of the Patella.

2   osteitis – Brodie's abcess

3   ant. tibial compartment syndrome

4   stress fracture

5   shin splints

6   plantaris tendon rupture

7   varacosities – tenderness – thrombophlebitis

8   Achille's tendon (tendocalcaneus) stress, tear or rupture

see also The knee - Extensor Apparatus

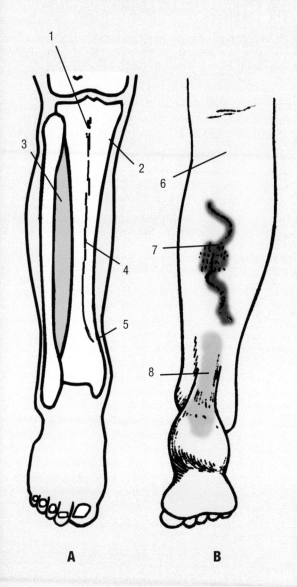

A

B

The Shoulder

Pattern of pathological presentation – *the shoulder is the major joint of the UL. It is inherently unstable and prone to dislocation & the effects of chronic If. Commonest cause of pain Is due to NR irritation in the cervical region – cervical spondylosis, which can occur at any age. Pain in the UL extremities can also originate from the shoulder. Other pathologies have a peak age presentation as demonstrated.*

OI – osteitis – due to Staphylococcal In   Common only in the young due to the active growing centres.

In – Infections due to TB or gonorrhoea   These present later particularly the latter, and further systemic symptoms should be Ix.

RD – recurrent dislocation   Defn – If the acromioclavicular & sternoclavicular jts dislocate, they often recur & remain unstable. The dislocation of the glenohumeral jt is generally inferiorly, where there is the least jt support, and originally occurs due to trauma (sports injuries are common), but once present is likely to recur.

DBD – decompression bone disease   Defn – in impingement diseases due to constant P from the rotator cuff muscles ± swollen bursae in glenohumeral movement, the underlying bone gradually becomes eroded.

CT – calcifying tendinitis   Defn – degenerative changes in the rotator cuff may result in deposition of calcium – and so ossification of the tendons – resulting in incapacitating sudden pain DD gout.

FS – Frozen shoulder AKA idiopathic adhesive capsulitis of the shoulder   Defn – a clinical syndrome of severely restricted shoulder movement due to the thickening of the jt capsule. It is generally painful & may be preceded by minimum trauma, which triggers a slow Clf process which slowly continues and results in the loss of shoulder function. Rotation is the primary movement affected.

RCT – rotator cuff tears   This condition is related to the previous condition and may be the preceding event. It is important to treat the resulting If thoroughly to stop the continued degenerative process, leading to FS.

OA – osteoarthritis   Particularly of the acromioclavicular jt, which can be seen with prominent lipping around the jt. It mainly restricts rotation of the shoulder.

RC – radionecrosis of the Clavicle   Defn – generally a 2° condition developing after radiotherapy of the breast – (eg for the Tx of breast cancer). A spontaneous degeneration of the clavicle results.

© A. L. Neill

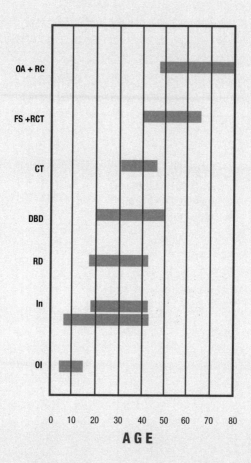

The Shoulder
Glenoid fossa anatomy

*The Gleno-humeral jt is the major jt of the shoulder
Its major articulating surface is the glenoid fossa of the
Scapula.*

*__Stability__ ++ - inherently unstable but reinforced by a
number of structures mainly surrounding the fossa.*

Together these form the shoulder cuff

*Schema   lat. view
            bony structures
            ligament supports
            other supports*

1 supraglenoid tubercle
2 coracoid process of the Scapula
3 glenoid – fossa is the depression in the centre

   3a = articular surface

4 tendon of long head of the biceps muscle
5 fibrocartilagenous labrium (lip) of the fossa
6 muscles – surrounding the shoulder – rotator cuff muscles

   6i = infraspinatus

   6s = supraspinatus

   6t = teres minor

   6u = subscapularis

7 joint capsule

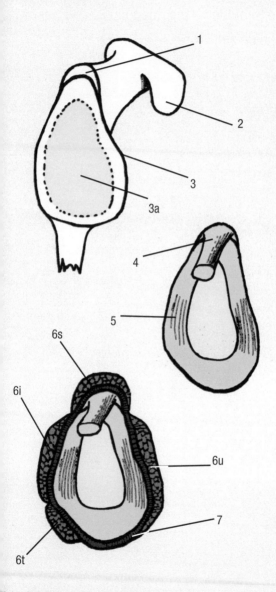

© A. L. Neill

The Shoulder - the Scapula
Dynamic Anatomy

The Scapula is a mobile structure
independent movements – not associated with arm
movements

D   depression

E   elevation
     range ~ 12cm

gleno-humeral associated movements – assisting arm
movements

L   lateral rotation

M   medial rotation

tD   tilting down

tU   tilting up
     range up to 60º

Note: the mobile scapula depends upon the mobility of the other shoulder jts

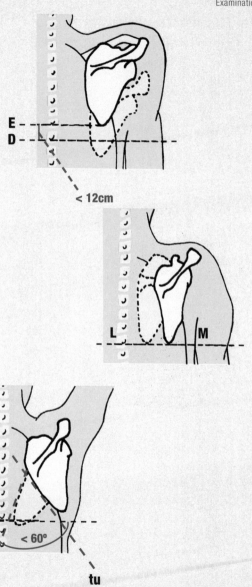

The Shoulder – radiology schema
Anatomical & Pathological features

Radiology views of shoulder

A A/P recumbency

B A/P features of the older shoulder

C A/P features of the younger shoulder

1 glenoid

2 lat. border of the Scapula

3 med. border of the Scapula

4 spine of the Scapula

5 Clavicle

6 acromion

7 coracoid process

8 ribcage underlying the shoulder

9 calcification of the suprspinatus tendon – appears as an amorphous mass – may be symptomless

10 "hatchet head" lesion – cause of recurrent dislocation because of bony distortion

11 OA of the acromioclavicular jt

12 inf. osteophytes of Humerus associated with rotator cuff pathology

13 exostosis on the inf. / costal surface of the Scapula assoc with shoulder clicking & snapping (lateral view shows this structure morel clearly

14 acromial ossification centre of the young shoulder

15 epiphyseal lines if the shoulder – not a fracture when seen in the young shoulder

16 ossifying chondroma – seen in young shoulders

** More details of the structure of the shoulder can be found in **The A to Z of the bones joints & ligaments and the Back***

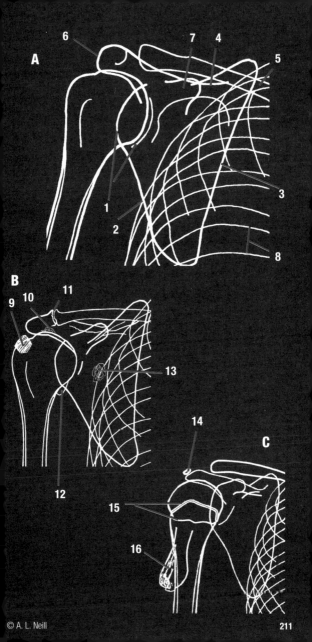

© A. L. Neill

The Shoulder
Inspection

Always compare with the normal side and observe the patient's posture for an overall assessment of the shoulder

A ant. view

B lat. view

C post. view

D superior view

1 Deltoid wasting – due to disuse, axillary N palsy

2 prominent acromioclavicular jt – DD OA or subluxation

3 deformity of the clavicle – DD previous #s

4 prominent sternoclavicular jt – DD subluxation

5 asymmetry of the supraclavicular fossa – DD due to Scapula displacement, muscle wasting

6 asymmetry of the nipples (6) DD posture & shoulder carriage changes, muscular asymmetry

7 swelling DD calcifying supraspinatus tendinitis, If, trauma.

8 high small Scapula – winged Scapula DD Kippel-Fiel syndrome, Sprengle's shoulder

9 neck webbing assoc with Scapula changes

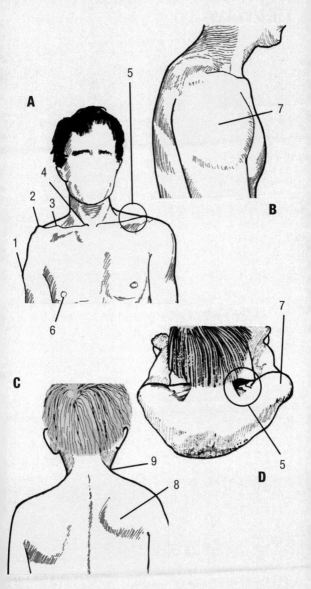

A

B

C

D

1
2
3
4
5
6
7
8
9

The Shoulder
Examination

A   General Instability – The Sulcus sign

The shoulder is fairly stable but has a deficiency inferiorly which may then extend & become a general instability. Hence a positive sign of inferior instability is a sign of a general instability.

Pull down on the relaxed arm of the standing patient & observe if a sulcus (1) develops. Compare with the normal side.

B   General joint pain

The shoulder has a number of articulations all of which may contribute to a generalized pain & restriction of movement.

Passively abduct the arm while palpating the jt & feeling for clicking &/or crepitus, repeat with active movement & note any difference in ROM. Clicking indicates: biceps tendon instability, coracoid impingement, rotator cuff instability &/or scapular exostoses. Crepitus indicates OA from either the acromioclavicular or glenohumeral jts.

A

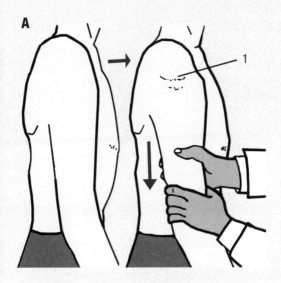

1

B

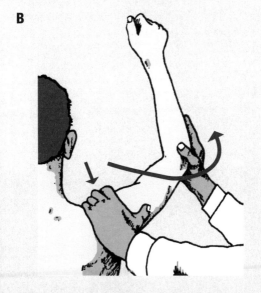

The Shoulder
Movements

The shoulder is capable of a number of complex movements but the following are good screening movements as they cannot be completed if there is any shoulder failure – in particular in the rotator cuff region.

A   post. view of arm internally rotated, adducted & flexed – if this can be completed the function of the shoulder is not seriously affected

B   post. view incomplete hand elevation on the back – ask for the hand to move off the back to see if scapularis is still intact – this is seen in the frozen shoulder

C   post. view – arm extended, abducted & extended – if this is symmetrical then the shoulder has reasonable function – not possible with a frozen shoulder

D   post. view – uneven movement – examiner to check the strength of this position will determine the strength of the shoulder

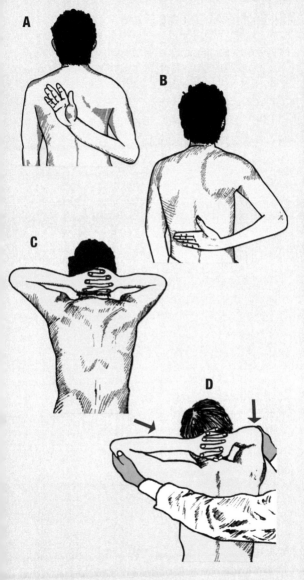

The Vertebral Column – the "Spine"

Anatomy – 9 articulations in the average vertebra: 2 upper & 2 lower zygoapophyseal jts – planar synovial jts: 1 upper & 1 lower symphysis VB to VB via fibrocartilagenous disc & 3 syndesmoses – connecting the spinous & transverse processes of each vertebra via ligs*, forming a long continuous flexible line of bone & ligs.

Stability – +++ - ++++ regionally varied The surfaces are compatible and are surrounded by a number of supporting ligs. & other bony structures eg ribs.

A   exploded diagram of the vertebral components – superiolat reconstructed components – superiolat

B   movements possible with the bony surfaces – lat

Bony components

1   Vertebral body (VB) – P weight bearing site of the VC – cancellous bone covered by a shell of compact bone

2   2 bony stems – allowing for articulation (2a) above & below with adjacent Vs (note the plane of this articulation varies regionally)

3   3 bony processes – 2 transverse & 1 spinous platforms for lig & muscle attachment & acting as bony shields around neural outflow

4   Bony neural arch – covering the SC – inserting into the articular pillars which divide it into 2 parts – the pedicle 4p & the lamina (wall) 4L

Neural components

5   SC

6   NR = nerve root spinal nerve – and foramen through which it emerges – made up of the 2 surrounding Vs

Disc components

7   Outer – annulus fibrosis – fibrocartilagenous ring

8   Inner – nucleus pulposis – gelatinous ring

Movements

9   Extension

10   Flexion

11   Lateral flexion – both ways mainly Lumbar region

12   Rotation – only in the thoracic region

© A. L. Neill

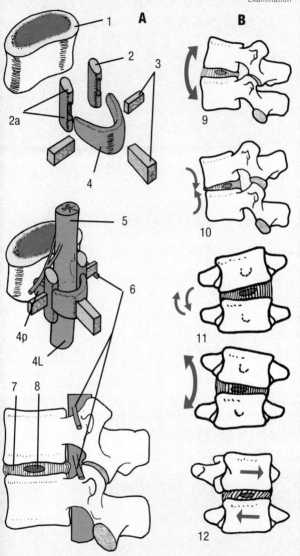

A   **B**

* More details of the structure of the VC / & specifically the "back" can bo
found in The A to Z of the Bones, Joints & Ligaments and the Back

© A. L. Neill

The Vertebral Column – the "Spine"

Prolapsed Disc Anatomy – Because of the structure of the intervertebral disc & the constant weightbearing – the central nucleus pulposis may herniate, through the annulus fibrosis or the VB, commonly called a "slipped disc".

A   posterior herniation – potentially impinges on the SC – bilateral symptoms in the legs ± bladder involvement

B   lateral herniation – potentially impinges on the SN – unilateral localized symptoms of the LL.

C   anterior herniation – into the VB – uncommon alters the VC curve

   central herniation – into the VBN – generally associated with other pathology weakening the bone structure e.g. OP seen in older patients

1   annulus fibrosis

2   nucleus pulposis (np)

3   np protrusion posteriorly into the vertebral canal

4   np protrusion posteriolaterally into the neural canal – outlet of the spinal Ns = NRs

5   SN = nerve root

6   np protrusion anteriorly

7   np breaking through the compact bone of the VB
   – pooling in the cancellous bone forming Scmorl's node

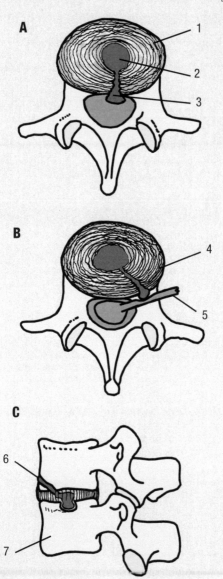

The Vertebral Column – radiology schema
Radiology views of the VC – Pathological features

A   Lateral view – normal thoracic curve

B   Lateral view – typical senile kyphosis

C   Lateral view – angular kyphosis

D   A/P view – scoliosis

E   Lateral view – normal lumbar curve

F   Lateral view – loss of lordosis

1   local VB collapse pathological # altering thoracic curve – seen post trauma, In, neoplasia, OP, osteomalacia.

2   point of jt space expansion in scoliosis

3   note the VB rotated towards the concavity jt space narrowing – (indicates cartilage loss)

4   rib distortion due to VC curving

5   loss of curvature does not result in bone distortion – & is often caused by reactive muscle contraction to reduce N pain from compressed VBs.

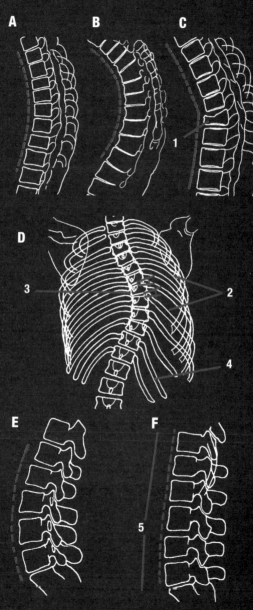

The Vertebral Column – radiology schema
Radiology views of the VC – Pathological features

A   Lateral view – Paget's disease

B   Lateral view – Calve's disease

C   Lateral view – space occupying lesions in VB

D   Lateral view – OA

1.   area of ⬆ density in VB with Picture frame border – seen in Paget's

2.   narrowing with ⬆ VB density – possible post crush # of VB – causing alteration of lumbar curve

3.   rounded VB due to erosions – as in early ankylosing spondylitis

4.   space occupying lesion in VB – In, Tm, Schmorl's node (as in collapsed VB)

5.   anterior lipping in chronic disc lesions

6.   jt space

7.   impingement of the SPs – "kissing spines" sign of collapsed disc space

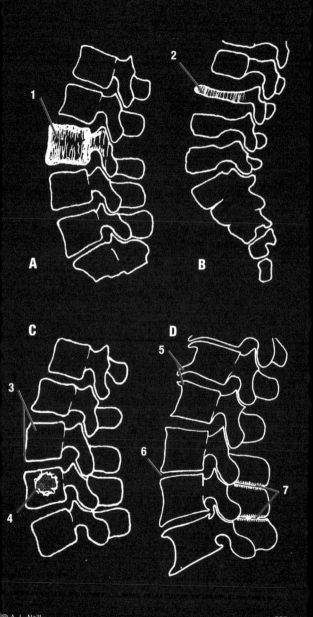

A

B

C

D

The Vertebral Column – radiology schema
Radiology views of the VC – Spondylolithesis

A   Lateral view – spondylolithesis
B   Lateral view – retrospondylolithesis
C   Oblique views – schema of features NAD
D   Oblique views – schema of features spondylolithesis

1   degree of VB slippage – f = fracture of the spinous process
    *Scotty dog – used to help in the identification of normal &
    abnormal features in the VC*
2   superior articular process
3   transverse process
4   pars interarticularis
5   inferior articular process
    Pathological changes in spondylolithesis
6   broken neck in forward spondylolithesis
7   near breakage from slipping – collar on the neck
8   early stages – elongation of the neck

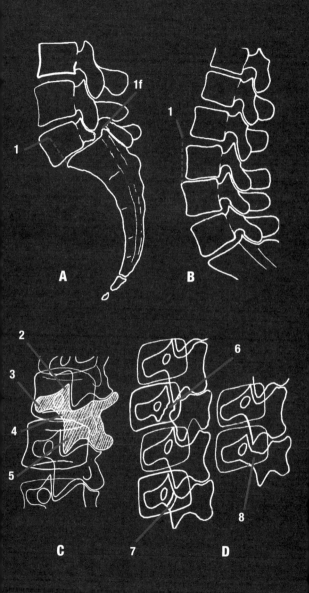

A

B

C

D

© A. L. Neill

Lucent Bone Lesions
X-ray detection of bone failure – due to radiolucent areas

When bone failure or pathology is detected one of the first tests to undertake is an X-ray. Results often show "lucent lesions" – areas in the bone where there is a localized decreased bone mass, which appears clearer on the X-ray. The site of these lesions – although they often appear similar – helps in the Dx of the bone pathology.

This is a guide of the aetiologies of these lucent areas in a typical LB.

Schema of LB – the Tibia

A   articulating surface

B   compact bone

BM bone marrow

CB cancellous bone

E   epiphysis

EP epiphyseal plate

M   metaphysis

1 Adamantinoma (rare)	9 Osteochondroma
2 Osteoid osteoma	10 Fibrous cortical defect
3 Chondromyxoid fibroma	11 Bone cyst
4 Osteosarcoma	12 Fibrosarcoma
5 Enchondroma	13 Fibrous dysplasia
6 Chondroblastoma '	14 "round cell lesions" e.g. Ewing's sarcoma, histiocytic lymphoma, myeloma
7 Giant cell tumour	
8 Aneurysmal bone cyst	

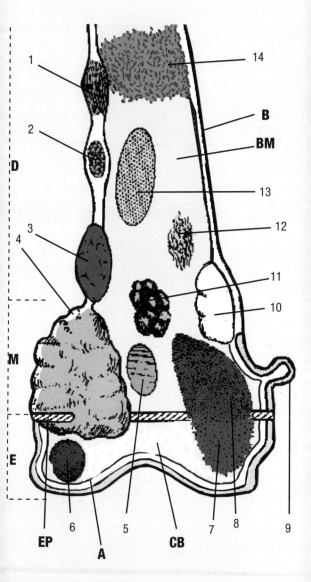

Necrosis – Cell / Tissue death
There are 4 main types of necrosis

I Caseous (Cheeselike)

Death due to a combination of lack of oxygen and a fatty degeneration common in TB Ins (II + IV)

Features – amorphous friable necrotic material is walled off by møs which form a surrounding epithelioid granuloma and giant cells

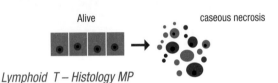

Alive   caseous necrosis

Lymphoid T – Histology MP

1. normal lymphoid T
2. epithelioid granuloma cells – transformed møs
3. giant cells (Langerhan's)
4. caseous necrosis

II Coagulative = Infarct

Death due to the sudden reduction / removal of BS – to a T or organ

Features sharply defined borders juxtaposed to an If region and then normal T

Renal T – Histology MP

1. ghost tubules – cells have died CT structure still preserved
2. coagulative necrosis – dead cells w/o membranes or structure – pool of cytoplasm & dead organelles
3. Inflammatory cells at the edge of the necrotic material
4. normal unaffected T

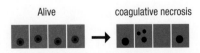

Alive   coagulative necrosis

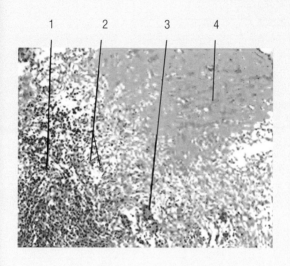

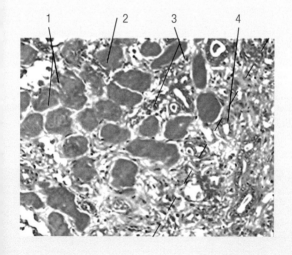

III Fat (+ Enzymatic)

Breast T – Histology MP

Death due to enzymatic digestion of fat T – large amounts of enzymes are released into the T & cause destruction – frequently post-traumatic.

Features – creamy firm focal deposits surrounded by IfR, generally occurs over osseous protuberances, unless generalized due to pancreatic death, gross release of enzymes.

Often difficult to demonstrate as the "fat" washes out in histological processing and the T appears "empty" – these holes are filled with the white creamy fat deposits described.

1   normal breast T
2   normal gland and tubules
3   large area of digestion – fat filled
4   swelling cells with digested contents and PMN infiltrate

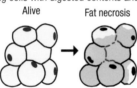

Alive   Fat necrosis

IV Liquefactive

Death due to the dissolution of the T & it becoming a fatty amorphous pool.

Often due to massive bacterial invasion which ruptures large numbers of cells with high fat content.

Brain T – Histology MP

1   Gliosis – in numbers of glial cells – these cells are the CT of the brain and they try to contain the pathological process
2   If zone of cells attracted to the dead T to try and "mop" it up and kill the causative agent
3   liquefactive necrosis – pool of amorphous fat
4   relatively normal unaffected T

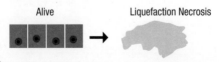

Alive   Liquefaction Necrosis

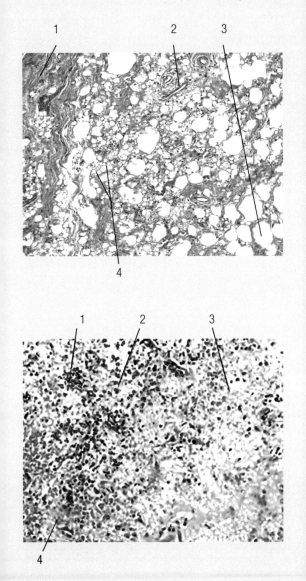

Osteogenesis Imperfecta = Brittle Bone syndrome

Osteogenesis Imperfecta (OI) is a rare genetic disease - with very fragile bones, causing the subject to have numerous fractures, due to poor collagen formation, particularly type 1 collagen. There are at least 2 forms of collagen in the body and 1 or both may be affected – so that the clinical picture varies considerably. There are several types with varying degrees of severity and morbidity and changes in the malformation of the collagen. These subgroups change, with new research findings.

A   schema of the collagen syntheses in OI

Collagen may be interrupted at various stages of its synthesis and the results will lead to a brittle bone type

1   transcription – most cases – have abnormal genes – so the fault is here

2   translation from DNA – to RNA

3   deposition of OH and glycoslate groups on the pro-collagen strand

4   assembly of pro-collagen strands & di-sulphide bonds

5   triple helix assembly of the collagen

6   protein suicide – this is seen in the severest forms of OI

7   assembly of the helix – but with aberrant proteins which shorten its life & alter its structure – this is seen in the less severe types

8   extrusion of collagen units – ready for final assembly in the fibre with an aberrant fibre structure the collagen fibril is not as strong & its weaker structure leads to weker shorter lasting bone T

B   schema comparing bones of normal vs OI

9   compact bone – thinner in the OI

10   trabeculae – fewer and thinner in OI

11   osteoid T laid down by the OBs is similar in both cases – but the bone laid down is not as stable

12   OCs / Giant cells more numerous in OI – due to the weakness of the bone laid down

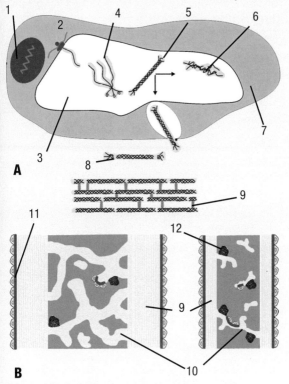

A

B

Type I	*Type II*
Commonest & mildest • bones # occur before puberty • normal stature • loose joints & muscle weakness • sclera usually have a blue, purple, or gray tint • triangular face • ± spinal curves • kyphosis &/or scoliosis • ± bone deformity • ±brittle teeth • ± hearing loss > 20yo • collagen structure is normal.	Most severe form • Frequently lethal at or shortly after birth, often due to respiratory problems • Numerous fractures and severe bone deformity, barrel chests • Small stature with underdeveloped lungs • Tinted sclera • Collagen improperly formed.

Spina Bifida

This disease presents as many different types – all with missing or incomplete vertebrae – generally in the lumbar or sacral regions. In Spina Bifida there may be no symptoms and it may be discovered on X-Ray. The hair over the defect is a sign & ⬆ LBP is associated with this – but in the more severe forms there may be debilitating functional deficiencies.

A   superior view of lumbar vertebrae in Spina Bifida

B   **Occulta** = hidden Outer part of the vertebrae are not completely joined but the SC & Meninges are intact and undamaged – Hair is often over the site of the defect.

C   **Meningocele** Outer part of the vertebrae split & the meninges are pushed to the surface

D   **Myelomeningocele** Spinal cord also pushed out – with possible hydrocephalus.

1	defect in the lumbar vertebrae – spine and laminae missing	4	dura mater
		5	vertebral body
		6	hair
2	skin	7	SC
3	arachnoid mater	8	subarachnoid space

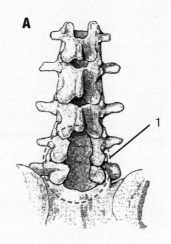

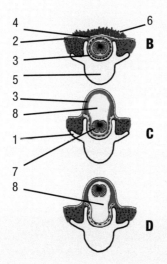

Osteomyelitis –
Haematogenous / Purulent

Infective organisms reach the metaphysis via the nutrient BVs of the bone. Once there, they proliferate & evoke the IR and abscess formation; leading to bone destruction. Further bacterial growth results in spread to the BM cavity & to the cortex. The purulent exudate lifts off the periosteum – cutting off the other nutrient BVs, which causes pathological #s so avascular bone is trapped inside the exudates & dies. The periosteum responds by sequestering FBs to form new bone outside the old bone line. After a cure this is remodelled to reform along the force lines.

Schema – progression of blood borne infection in LB (Tibia)

1 compact bone + EP

2 medullary cavity – site of red BM

3 medullary cavity site of yellow BM

4 site of In introduced via the ...

5 nutrient BVs

6 periosteum

7 abscess formation + spread to other cavities

8 lifting of the periosteum – shearing off the nutrient BVs

9 adjacent bone reacting to bacterial In and IR

10 sinus – escape of purulent exudates out of the bone

11 pathological # resulting in trapped avascular bone fragments = sequestra

12 reactive bone – involucrum – a layer of new bone formation stimulated by sequestration of fibroblasts from the periosteum

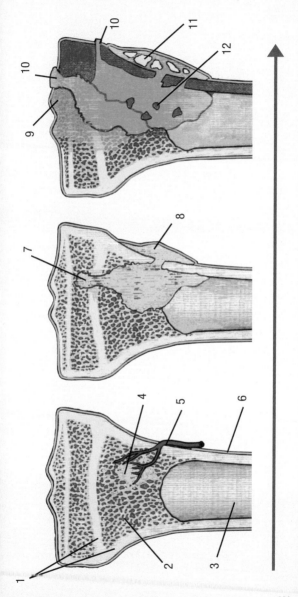

© A. L. Neill

Osteoarthritis (OA) vs Rheumatoid Arthritis (RA)

Arthritis = joint inflammation – This can be due to wear and tear OA or to other factors including autoimmune factors as seen in RA.

Schema – OA joint
– RA joint

1 bone cyst

2 joint capsule

3 synovial membrane

4 osteophyte – overgrowth of bone due to joint breakdown

5 EP

6 bone erosion = w/o covering articular cartilage due to wear and tear from unequal forces

6p bone erosion due to Pannus overgrowth

7 pannus = inflammatory overgrowth of synovial membrane

8 articular cartilage

9 joint space – note this is narrowed in both diagrams compared to a normal joint

10 BM

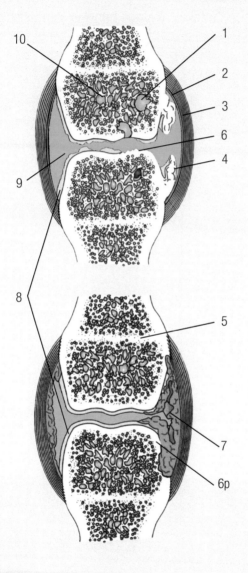

Biomechanics of weight-bearing joints

Normal synovial joint undergoes deformation when weight bearing to disperse the load. If this does not happen then weight is not dissipated but concentrated on the edges of the joint, eventually loading to its breakdown – and development of osteoarthritis (OA).

Schema – normal joint
– abnormal joint

F   weight-bearing force down on the joint

DF dispersed force

CF concentrated force

AC articular cartilage surface

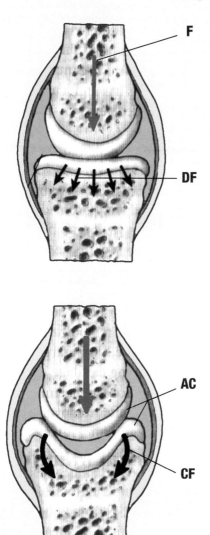

Calcium Regulation

Bone T is an important store of Calcium (Ca). The parathyroid glands – 4 small bean shaped organs buried in the posterior of the thyroid gland are the main controls of the serum Ca levels, via Parathyroid Hormone (PH). The thyroid gland parafollicular cells secrete Calcitonin which is weaker and antagonizes PH. Ca is essential for: blood clotting, enzyme activation & regulation, heart beat regulation, muscle contraction & relaxation and N impulse transmissions. It makes up 2% of the body weight most of which is in the skeleton & teeth.

A ○ extracellular concentrations of Ca ↓

B causing the parathyroid glands to signal serum Ca preservation by secreting PH

which causes:

CA – absorption of Ca from the GIT

CB – release of Ca from bone

CR re-absorption of Ca from the kidney with excretion of PO_4^{3-}

A ● ↑ extracellular concentrations of Ca ↑

B causing the thyroid gland – parafollicular cells to signal serum Ca to ↓ via Calcitonin encouraging bone formation –

CA is blocked

CB is blocked

CR is blocked

1 thyroid gland
2 parathyroid gland
3 kidney + ureter
4 GIT
5 bone
6 extracellular fluids

© A. L. Neill

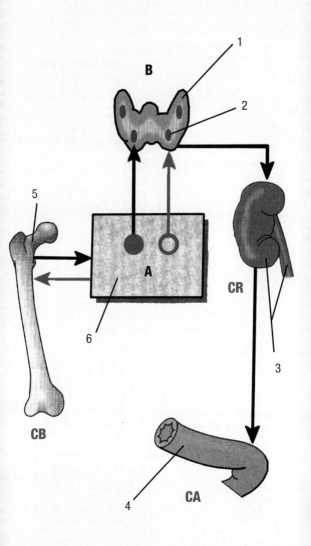

Calcium & Phosphate Regulation

Bone T is an important store of Calcium (Ca), which is linked to Phosphate (PO). The parathyroid glands are sensitive to both the serum levels of Ca & PO S(Ca) and high levels of S(PO) may cause the elimination of Ca from the body. Both ions are in balance, Ca x PO = Z. Because of the neuromuscular Ca S(Ca) must be maintained w/n a strict range, even at the cost of bone strength.

Calcium (Ca) & Phosphate (PO) both need Vitamin C & D to allow for their absorption, secretion & serum levels.

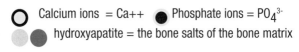

Calcium ions = Ca++   Phosphate ions = PO_4^{3-}

hydroxyapatite = the bone salts of the bone matrix

1   parathyroid glands
2   thyroid gland
3   PH pathway
4   Ca & PO normally diffuse across the renal tubules
5   PH – causes Ca to be reabsorbed but inhibits PO
6   remaining Ca & PO lost in the urine
7   bone matrix + hydroxyapatite – OCs ⬆
8   Vitamin C + acidity ⬆
9   OCs
10 Normally bone formation (bf)= resorption (bs) bf>bs growth / bf<bs OP

11 OB (laying down bone)
12 B-AP ⬆ with bone formation
13 S(Ca) ⬇ S(PO) ⬇ – move into bone
14 blood pH – acidity favours blood Ca ⬆ (out of bone) – alkalinity favours blood Ca ⬇ & PO ⬇ (into bone)
15 GIT secretions – including bile / stomach acid / pancreatic enzymes facilitate
16 Vitamin D to absorb Ca & PO across the gut
17 Cortisol opposes the action of Vitamin D
18 Ca / PO balance directly affects the PH levels – both high levels of Ca or PO ⬇ PH – low levels of Ca ⬆ PH

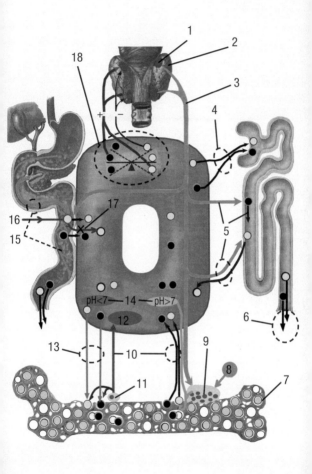

pH<7 — 14 — pH>7

Parathyroid glands – in situ

The parathyroid glands are 4 (range 3-6) small beanlike mustard coloured endocrine glands which are embedded in the back of the thyroid gland surrounding the trachea (hence the name – "near" the thyroid), normal size b/n 30-200 mg 5x5x5mm. Adenomas grow up to 500mg. They act independently of the thyroid, and are responsible for the Calcium (Ca) & Phosphate (P) levels in the body via the Parathyroid hormone (PH). PH works on a feedback loop – stimulating Ca to be mobilized from bone and other areas if the serum levels are low, but they have no direct effect on OBs & so do not effect the laying down of bone.

Constant high levels of the H result in excessive Ca mobilization from bone, weakening it & causing OP.

1   Parathyroid gland
2   Thyroid gland
3   BVs
4   Capsule of parathyroid
5   Chief cells – responsible for the production of PH – main cells
6   Oxyphil cells ? function unknown – do not appear until > 5yo ⬆ with age. They are large acid-loving cells, clustered in groups.

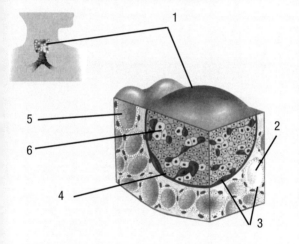

Calcium & Phosphate Regulation
Hyperparathyroidism & Osteitis Fibrosa Cystica (OFC)

Bone T is an important store of Calcium (Ca), which is linked to Phosphate (PO), in an inverse relationship – primarily controlled by PH. In hyperparathyroidism – OFC develops. Irregular bone density, ⬆ bone cycle leads to strong trabeculae being replaced by weaker fibrous T & cysts. ⬆ Pathological #s occur bc of poor bone, stones form in the kidney bc of ⬆ u (Ca) along with ⬆ nausea & ⬆ anorexia.

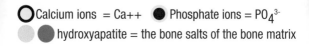

⭕ Calcium ions = Ca++   ⚫ Phosphate ions = PO_4^{3-}

🔵⚫ hydroxyapatite = the bone salts of the bone matrix

1   parathyroid glands with hyperparathyroidism due to:
a = adenoma – 80% / b = clear cell hyperplasia – 10% / c = chief cell hyperplasia – 8% / d = carcinoma of the parathyroid gland – 2%

2   thyroid gland

3   PH pathway – ⬆ due to hyperparathyroidism & causing

     4   ⬆ serum levels of Ca – but low PO levels

     5   ⬆ levels of Ca are excreted via the kidney due to the high serum levels

     6   ⬆ PO levels are excreted via the kidney because resorption is blocked via the PH

Leading to the formation of renal stones (7)

8   PH – ⬆ OCs to resorb bone causing

9   bone cysts ("brown" tumours) – pathological #s

10   irregular bone density develops – partic subperiosteal resorption & fibrous replacement from irregular OC stimulation & irregular OB stimulation

11   OB – laying down additional bone in response to the resorption & ⬆ serum Ca

12   B-AP ⬆ with bone formation

13   PH causes ⬆ Ca & PO absorption from the GIT so …

     14   ⬆ movement to the bone

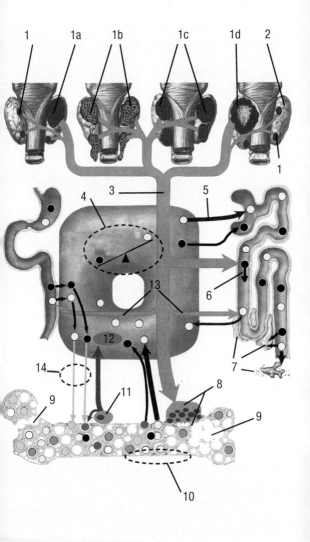

Calcium & Phosphate Regulation
Hypoparathyroidism

Bone T is an important store of Calcium (Ca), which is linked to Phosphate (PO), in an inverse relationship – primarily controlled by the parathyroid gland. When the parathyroid glands are absent via surgery (accidental removal with thyroidectomy), congenital absence – or chemical shutdown, the bone is affected adversely.

Serum PO levels rise because PH is not present there to stop PO resorption. OCs ⬇ Ca mobilization from bone ⬇ but bone continues to be formed at the normal rate. However the serum Ca is lower & this affects its other roles in the body.

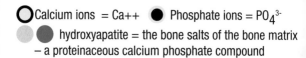

⬤ Calcium ions $= Ca++$ ⬤ Phosphate ions $= PO_4^{3-}$

⬤⬤ hydroxyapatite = the bone salts of the bone matrix
– a proteinaceous calcium phosphate compound

1   parathyroid glands absent due to surgery (a) or other rare causes (b) eg congenital.

2   Ca – PO balance – PO ⬆ and Ca reduced

3   PH pathway – absent due to lack of glands

    4 Ca absorption from the GIT ⬇ – no PH

    5 Ca absorption from the GIT ⬇ binds to the ⬆ PO

6   urine Ca ⬇ because of the low serum levels

7   urine PO ⬇ it is actively resorbed from the kidneys no PH to block it

8   OCs ⬇ Ca & PO not mobilized and bone turnover is ⬇ no PH

9   OBs continue unaffected by the loss of PH – laying down new bone

10 bone density ⬆

11 Alkaline phosphatase unaffected

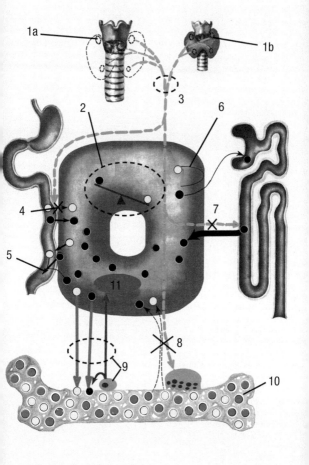

Osteomalacia (& Rickets – children)

Osteomalacia (OM) is UNDERMINERALIZATION of the bone matrix, due to ⬇ serum Ca.

Causes of which are:

⬇ *Vitamin D, associated with fat malabsorption (2) &/or ⬇ sunlight (3);*

⬆ *dietary PO or phytates (4) which ⬇ GIT Ca absorption (5);*

⬆ *demands for Ca as in pregnancy or lactation (6) or excessive sweating*

⬇ *re-absorption of Ca from the kidney in the DCT (7) – renal osteodystrophy.*

Low serum Ca (1) feeds back (10) to the parathyroid gland (8) & ⬆ PTH levels (9); hence PO reabsorption is ⬇ across the renal tubules (11) so then both serum Ca & PO are reduced (12). Ca & PO are both mobilized from the bone – via the OCs (13), but do not leave the serum to form new bone (14) – even though the OBs (15) are stimulated by the weakened bone & form more & more bone, which is poorly formed & undermineralized (16). This weak bone develops irregular lucent areas of bone – (17) Looser's lines or bodies AKA pseudofractures AKA Milkman's syndrome & moth-eaten EPs in immature bones (18). OBs lay down excessive osteoid T seams beneath the periosteum (19) & this leads to ⬆ BVs (20) & fibrous T in the bone T - flattening & broadening of bones in the adult (OM) & bending of the LBs in the child (Rickets). Bone turnover is ⬆ so Alkaline phosphatase (21) is ⬆.

Typical features are similar to those of Paget's disease:

Flat occiput, frontal bossing & square head

Overgrowth of cartilage at costochondral junctions

Pigeon chest

Harrison's sulcus

Lumbar lordosis

Leg bowing

The bone is prone to #s – particularly the VBs & NOF

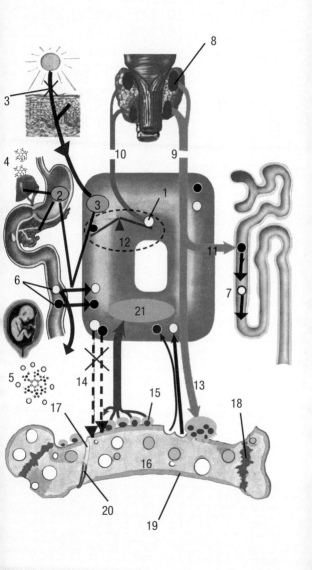

Differential Diagnoses of Hypercalcaemia

Condition	Calcium Blood levels	Urine levels	Phosphate Blood levels	Alkaline Phosphatase (Indicates bone metabolism ▲)	OTHER FINDINGS
1° Carcinoma – not bone	◄	◄	▼◄	▢	lung cancer bronchogenic
Carcinoma – 2° to bone	◄	◄	■◄	▣◄	Lucent X-ray lesions
Disuse atrophy Long standing Immobilization	◄	◄	■◄	■	DD OP
Hyperparathyroidism	◄	◄	▶	■◄	sub-periosteal resorption
Milk Alkali syndrome	◄	▶	■	■	alkalosis / ulcer Hx / subcutaneous calcification
Multiple myeloma	◄	◄	■	■◄	Bence – Jones proteins in urine ▲ / serum globulin levels ▲
Sarcoidosis	◄	◄	■◄	■◄	serum globulin levels ▲
Thyrotoxicosis	◄	◄	■◄	■◄	weight loss / hyperactivity
Hypervitaminosis – D	◄	◄	■◄	■	Hx of Vitamin D ingestion

Osteoporosis
Common sites of Fractures

Because of the lower bone mass in OP – it is more likely to fracture, either after a fall or causing a fall.

The commonest sites are

1 the VC – particularly in the thoracic region develops pathological fractures in the VBs – and ⬆ the normal thoracic curve – kyphosis – forming a dowager's hump. In the lumbar region this can lead to N compression and sciatic pain

2 the NOF is very vulnerable partic with a fall to fracture

3 when falling, arm is often extended & broken at the wrist Colle's fracture

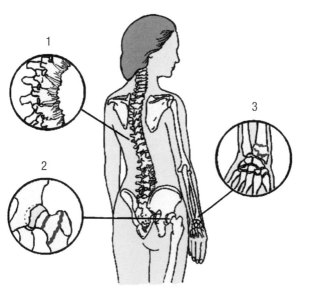

Osteoporosis –
Hip Joint Pelvic girdle + Femur

Osteoporosis is a "poverty" of bone AKA smooth bone atrophy. It cannot be detected until 30% bone mass has been lost, and is often picked up when the bone "fails" by fracturing under the weight it can no longer support. Hence weight bearing bones & joints are most at risk – such as the Femur. A broken "hip" from a small trauma – or none at all in the elderly female is a typical presentation.

Bone T which is constantly remodelling – becomes unbalanced in that the "clastic" or phagocytic activity > the "blastic" or new bone formation. Hence total bone mass is reduced.

Cortical bone & cancellous bone are both lost. It is reversible, in the early stages – trabeculae can be rebuilt and cortical bone thickened – but trabeculae cannot be reformed once gone.

Macro of the Head of the Femur and Pelvic girdle
A NAD
B OP

1 head of Femur
2 neck of Femur
3 cortical bone
4 normal cancellous bone
   m = magnified
5 BM cavity
6 thinner fewer bone trabeculae
   m = magnified
7 thinner cortical bone
8 "hip" joint
9 sites of weakness & possible pathological fractures

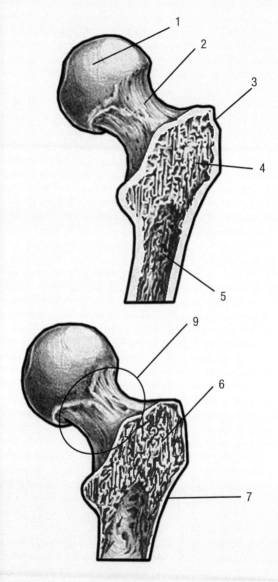

A

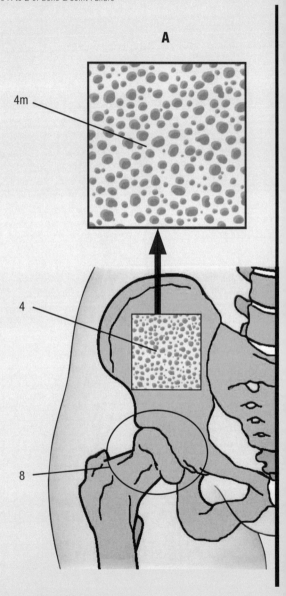

4m

4

8

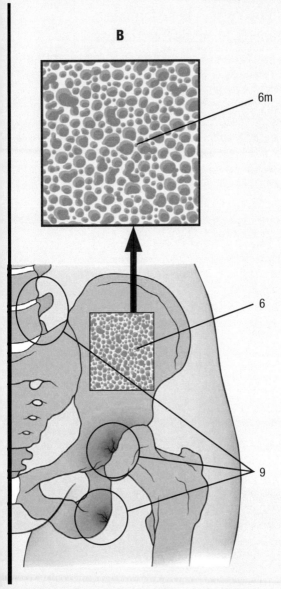

B

6m

6

9

Osteoporosis & Bone formation
Vitamins, Minerals & Hormones

Bone is constantly forming & reforming throughout life. It is one of the T in the body with the highest metabolism & so is sensitive to dietary, hormonal & lifestyle changes. It requires a number of inter-related substances & conditions to form correctly. The deficiency or excess of any can lead to serious bone malformation. Listed below are substances implicated in bone development & OP. This list is not complete & does not list substances for which there is no clear relationship b/n bone & OP. Other substances may be involved in the development of OP. These include alcohol, caffeine & smoking.

Calcitonin – While PTH is the major H to control Ca metabolism – its weaker antagonist is Calcitonin derived from the parafollicular cells of the thyroid.

Calcium (Ca) – Normal bone is made up of 20% Ca. High dietary intakes of Ca alone will not stop bone loss with age & disuse. Dietary Ca needs to be in a form able to be absorbed from the GIT. Without fat in the diet it cannot be absorbed. High levels of dietary PO & phytates will ⬇ the amount of Ca absorbed. High levels of fruit, vegetables, and other alkaline substances will ⬇ the amount of Ca absorbed across the GIT – however the alkalinity is protective of bone Ca. High levels of protein and other acid substances will ⬆ the amount of Ca absorbed across the GIT, reabsorbed from the renal tubules & mobilized from bone.

Fluoride – The fluoride anion competes with other anions for a place in the bone T, mainly the PO. It leads to the deposition of more bone it is harder and brittle and may be more prone to # in osteopenic bones

Magnesium (Mg) – Mg makes up 0.1% of bone - & competes with other metal cations for transport in the GIT & renal reabsorption. Converts Vitamin D into its active form – w/o Mg Vitamin D is inactive. Fixes Ca onto collagen fibrils.

Metal cations e.g. Boron (B), Chromium (Cr), Copper (Cu), Magnesium (Mg), Manganese (Mn), Zinc (Zn)

Many metal cations compete for the same transport systems in the GIT & renal re-absorption. Too high levels of one will stop the adequate absorption of the others. B assists Ca, PO & Mg also ⬆ oestrogen & testosterone levels when in low levels – particularly important in the older patient both ♀ & ♂. Cr is involved with insulin activation & so may be implicated in DM type II OP. Cu & Mg are needed for CT formation. Cu is involved in antioxidant activity. Mn has antioxidant properties and prevent bone erosion by free radicals. Zn is necessary for bone formation particularly growing bones. It is thought necessary to attach the Ca to the bone matrix.

Oestrogen – ⬇ rate of bone turnover and preserves bone. ⬇ OC activity & other lf activity

Phosphorous / phosphate (PO) – Should be in the ratio of Ca:PO – 2:1 to 4:1 for a correct balance to be achieved – Ca will be robbed from bones to keep this balance. PTH promotes Ca GIT absorption & keeps the renal resorption of PO low to maintain this balance.

Silicon – This element is in the body in low levels and contributes to the strength of bone by inclusion in newly laid down bone.

Testosterone – This H may have a similar but less important role in maintaining total bone mass as oestrogen.

Vitamin A – Like the other fat soluble vitamins – D, E & K helps with the absorption of Ca across the GIT.

Vitamin C – Vitamin C is essential for the formation of collagen fibres w/o which there is no framework for the formation of bone

Vitamin D – Vitamin D is necessary for the absorption of Ca across the GIT, after being converted to its active form.

Osteoporosis & Osteopenia
Peak Bone Mass

Bone is laid down from birth in a predictable pattern until it reaches a peak 25-35yo. This Peak Bone Mass – (PBM) is the point where bone is at its strongest. After this point it gradually declines. In men this continues into old age. In women it is further increased at menopause where the rate of bone loss is increased for about 10 yrs when it slows to decrease in the slower slope of old age.

At a critical point – the bone is below the normal range – OSTEOPENIA. Further decreases place the bone in the range of OSTEOPOROSIS & below that in the FRACTURE VULNERABLE range.

A   schema of bone growth in the female with optimal & suboptimal conditions

B   schema comparing bone mass density in ♂ versus ♀ in similar conditions

   1   threshold of normal bone mass

   2   threshold of the fracture vulnerability below which is irreversible bone loss – osteoporotic zone

      1-2 zone of osteopenia – reversible bone loss

   3   graph – of ♀ bone mass – under optimal lifestyle and nutritional conditions

   4   graph – of ♀ bone mass – until poorer conditions – vitamin deficencies etc

   5   graph of normal ♂ bone mass changes with age

   6   graph of normal ♀ bone mass changes with age

   7   PBM

   8   accelerated bone loss with menopause

   9   bone loss with age

  10   falls in the elderly much more likely to fracture / pathological fractures cause falls in the elderly

A

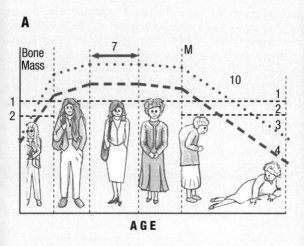

B

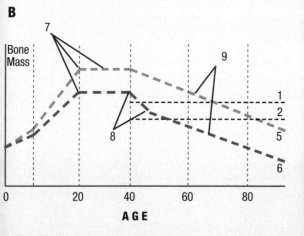

Paget's disease = Osteitis Deformans

Paget's disease is an idiopathic disease of the bone – showing an abnormal rapid formation of bone thicker but softer and deformed – affecting either only 1 bone – MONOSTOTIC in 1/3 of cases or many POLYOSTOTIC in 2/3 of cases. It is possibly a reaction to a viral disease (?).

incidence ~90% > 55yrs and rare < 40yrs ♂ > ♀ predominantly European

Sites	% involved	clinical changes
Femur	30%	bowing + #s
Lumbar spine	30%	crush # of the VBs / wedging
Pelvis	20%	hip dislocations
Ribs + thoracic VC	10%	kyphosis – VB #s
Skull	30%	enlargement – forehead bossing (6) / cranial exits stenosed
eyes		blindness – CN II compressed (4)
ears		deafness – CN VIII compressed (5)
Sternum	20%	warm – note the heart beat & CO is ⬆ (1)
Tibia	10%	bowing + #s + warmth over bones (2)

Whole body metabolism is ⬆ because of the rapid bone turnover.

Most weight bearing bones develop an arthritis as the bone softens and the jts are compromised – feet flatten and toes spread (3)

Px is poor – degeneration continues

Cancerous change is rare

© A. L. Neill

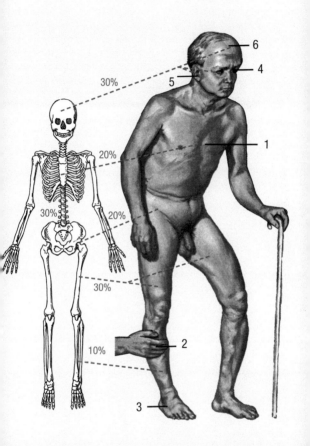

30%

20%

30% 20%

30%

10%

6

4

5

1

2

3

Paget's disease = Osteitis Deformans

Histological & Radiological changes

Paget's disease is an idiopathic disease of the bone. It is degenerative, growing through 3 main stages of deterioration which weakens and enlarges the bone but reduces its strength. This is the case in the monostotic localized and generalized forms of the disease.

Radiological changes

Early radiolucency w/o thickening of the bone (osteoporosis circumscripta)

Later ⬆ density with thick, coarse trabeculae, but cortical bone is weaker; there is loss of cortico-medullary demarcation – typical microfractures develop in the thickened bone.

Histological changes

A **Osteolytic phase** ⬆ GCs (1) resorption, ⬆ vascularity Trabeculae slender (2) & sparse in medulla (3) Resorption cavities in the cortical bone- lytic weak regions (4) Appositional new bone formation with prominent OBs (5) GCs generally larger & more numerous than seen in hyperparathyroidism

B **Osteoblastic phase** bone formation ⬆ Massive trabecular plates with a density that is neither cortical nor cancellous ⬆ number of reversal lines mosaic pattern of bone (6) – loss of Haversian osteons (7) ⬇ bone strength ➡ + cracks on the cortical bone – best seen with polarised light microscopy

C **Burnt out phase** ⬇ cellular activity, ⬇ vascularity ⬆ mosaic pattern BM may return to normal appearance – or remain reduced filled with abnormal bone ⬆ AP but Ca & P serum levels are normal

#s - neck femur & wedging of VBs
⬆ Arthritis ⬆ periosteal bone formation – so enlarged weak bones ⬆ bone cancers – sarcomas

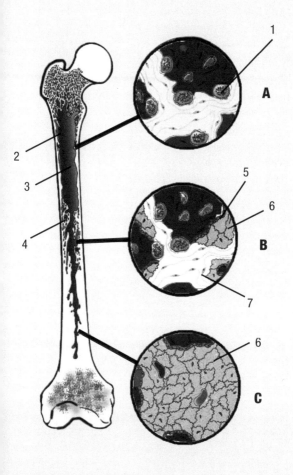

Avascular necrosis
AKA Aseptic necrosis AKA Osteonecrosis
AKA Bone infarct

Avascular necrosis is the bone necrosis due to the cessation of the BS to the bone – or joint. It can occur to any jt and frequently occurs in multiple jts – 2° to other diseases, or trauma but in many cases it is idiopathic.

Common sites are:

Femoral condyles, head	*hip jt = Perthes disease*
Humeral head	*knee jt, Tibial plateau*
Lunate Scaphoid wrist jt	*Shoulder jt*
Talus	

The articular cartilage is left w/o a BS and is decimated and flakes off Osteochondritis Dessicans

Pathogenesis

The necrotic bone & surrounding BM causes oedema, further venous obstruction and so a widening of the infracted area, further loss of function and ⬆ pain.

Radiological changes

Stage	Pain	Radiographs	Pathology
I	none	⬆ density of necrotic bone	creeping substitution
II	none	reactive rim in surrounding bones	rim, re-infarction
III	occasionally	crescent sign	fracture – just below jt surface
IV	limp, because of ⬇ weight bearing capacity, ⬇ function & ROM	step or flattening	loose fragments in jt space
V	continuous	collapse	cartilage flaps and flakes
VI	severe	deformed jt	advanced arthritis

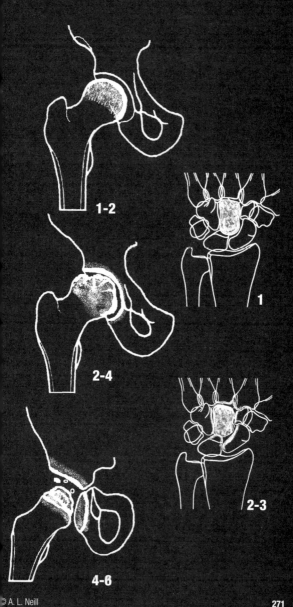

1-2

2-4

4-6

1

2-3

Common sites of Primary Malignant Neoplasms of bone

There are 4 common types of primary bone malignant cancers derived from the major cell types which make up bone T – most are relatively rare but they are essentially diseases of the young – making up 5% of all the cancers in children

Schema – sites of primary bone cancers

Chondosarcoma = tumour of the chondroblasts – cartilage forming bones

Aetiology – unknown
Incidence – 30% of all skeletal tumours – mainly older groups >50yo – likely to recur
Presenting SS – bone pain in the back or thigh ± sciatica & bladder symptoms ± oedema

Ewings sarcoma = small round (blue) cell tumour essentially a tumour of the BM cells

Aetiology – chromosomal translocation in many cases – genetic
Incidence – males > females 1.6:1 10-20yo   rare < 1:1,000,000
Presenting SS – localized bone pain ± swelling

Giant-cell tumour = tumour of the osteoclasts – multinucleated phagocytic bone cells

Aetiology – unknown
Incidence – females > males 1.2 > 1 20-30yo rare 4% of all skeletal tumours – likely to recur
Presenting SS – pathological #

Osteosarcoma = tumour of the osteoblasts
Aetiology – familial, radiotherapy, fluoridation of the water supply
Incidence – 20% of all bone cancers – peaks <20yo and then >50yo – generally aggressive with metatstoses – likely to recur
Presenting SS – localized but variable pain ± swelling ± pathological #

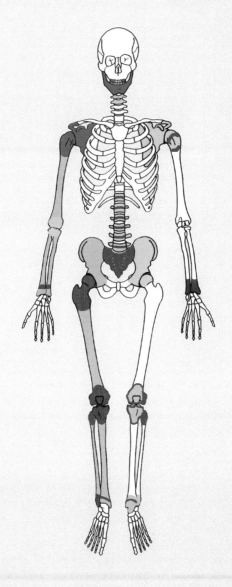

Lesion	Patient profile age	M:F	Bones in order of frequency -greatest to least	Location in the bone	features / Xray appearance location	Microscopic features	Behaviour
Osteoma	40-50	2:1	Skull & facial bones	-	may protrude inside a paranasal sinus	dense mature lamelar bone	benign
Osteoid osteoma	10-30	2:1	Femur, Tibia, Humerus, hands & feet, Vertebrae, fibula	cortex of M in LB	lucent central nidus <15mm± dense centre, peripheral sclerotic reaction; painful	sharply delineated nidus: osteoid lined by plump OBs; w/o lf	benign
Osteoblastoma	10-30	2:1	VBs, Tibia, Femur, Humerus, Pelvis, Ribs	medulla of M in LBs	larger nidus, absent reactive bone; not painful	aa	benign
Osteosarcoma	10-25	3:2	Femur, Tibia, Humerus, Pelvis, Jaw, Fibula	medulla of M in LBs	Codman's ▲; mets to lung/bone/ pleura/heart	osteoid produced by Tm cells w/o intervening cartilage	20% 5yr survival
Chondroma	10-40	1:1	hands & feet, Ribs, Femur, Humerus	medulla of D in LBs	enchondroma: begins in spongiosa of D, expands & thins cortex	mature lobules of cartilage	benign
Osteochondroma	10-30	1:1	Femur, Tibia, Humerus, Pelvis	cortex of M in LBs	grows out opposite to adj jt	cap of cartilage covered by a membrane continuous with periosteum	benign
Chondroblastoma	10-25	2:1	Femur, Humerus, Tibia, feet, Pelvis, Scapula	E	well delimited, areas of rarefaction; painful	extreme cellularity & variability, polyhedral cells, GC, glycogen, reticulin	benign
Chondromyxoid fibroma	10-25	1:1	Tibia, Femur, feet, Pelvis	M	sharply defined, may be large	hypocellular lobules with intersecting bands spind/OC	benign

Lesion	Patient profile age	M:F	Bones in order of frequency -greatest to least	Location in the bone	features / Xray appearance location	Microscopic features	Behaviour
Chondrosarcoma	30-60	3:1	Pelvis, Ribs, Femur, Humerus, VBs	cortex of M in LBs medulla of central bones	osteolytic with splotchy calcification	range of differentiation: cartilaginous matrix, lack of direct bone formation	low 78% / mod 53% / high 22% / 5 yr survival
Mesenchymal chondrosarcoma	20-60	1:1	Ribs, Skull, Mandible, VBs, Pelvis, soft tissues	D in LBs	aa	dimorphic: well-diff cartilage with undifferentiated stroma	v poor prognosis
Giant cell tumour	20-40	4:5	Femur, Tibia, Radius	E, M	lytic expansile lesion without sclerosis or a periosteal reaction	stromal cells, GCs	50% recur, 10% metastasize
Ewings sarcoma/ PNET	5-20	1:2	Femur, Pelvis, Tibia, Humerus, Ribs, Fibula;	medulla of D & M in LBs	cortical thickening with widening of the medullary canal; react periost	sheets of cells with fibrous strands, pseudorosettes, glycogen	20-30% 5 yr survival mets to lung, pleura, other bones
1° LCL, mixed cell types	30-60	1:1	Femur, Pelvis, VBs, Tibia, Humerus, Mandible, Skull, Ribs	medulla of D & M in LBs	bone production & destruction over a wide area	as per lymphoma elsewhere	22-50% 5 yr survival

The A to Z of Bone & Joint Failure

Lesion	Patient profile age	M:F	Bones in order of frequency - greatest to least	Location in the bone	features / Xray appearance location	Microscopic features	Behaviour
Plasma cell myeloma	40-60	2:1	VBs, Pelvis, Ribs, Sternum, Skull	medulla of E, D & M in LBs			diffuse always fatal
Heamangioma	20-50	1:1	Skull, VBs, Mandible	medulla	sunburst trabeculation 2° to periosteal elevation	thick walled lattice pattern of cavernous spaces	benign
Desmoplastic fibroma	20-30	1:1	Humerus, Tibia, Pelvis, Mandible, Femur, Scapula	M	lytic / honeycombed	mature fibroblasts, abundant collagen	benign
Fibrosarcoma	20-60	1:1	Femur, Tibia, Mandible, Humerus	medulla of M in LBs	osteolytic "soap-bubble"	as per soft T, no Tm osteoid	28% 5yr survival
Chordoma	40-60	2:1	Sacrococcygeal, Spheno-occipital, Cervical VBs	-	osteolytic, rarely osteoblastic	cords & lobules; physaliferous cells	malignant, 48% mets
Solitary bone cyst	10-20	3:1	Humerus, Femur	medulla of M	thin cortex		benign

276

© A. L. Neill

Appendix
Bone Diseases – their names & aetiologies

BONE & JOINT FAILURE

■ **congenital / genetic**

■ **idiopathic**

■ **inflammatory**

■ infective

■ **metabolic / iatrogenic or drug induced**

■ neoplastic

■ **trauma / mechanical / neuromuscular**

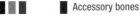 **Accessory bones**

These additional bones can occur anywhere – DD avulsed bone fragments and foreign bodies in jts as in the knee – occur in sites of strong tendons – and may be due to calcium being laid down in these areas.

of the foot

It is common to see additional bones in the foot – particularly around the Hallux, and near the Achilles tendon

■ **Achondroplasia (dwarfism)**

Genetic disorder of the LBs so the limbs are short but the head and other bones are of normal length. Commonest form is a genetic disease – dominant inheritance *see Hand examination*

■ ■ **Acromegaly** *see hyperpituitarism*

Adult form of Giantism – forming after the LBs have fused – so only the areas of bone with cartilage coverings can ⬆ – due to an excess of growth H

■ **Adhesive capsulitis** *see frozen shoulder*

With calcification in the capsular ligaments in reactive arthropathies and – heterotropic bone formation around jt replacements the capsule becomes fixed in the shoulder – 1st movement to be lost is rotational.

■ **Adolescent kyphosis** *see kyphosis*

■ **Alkaptonuria** *see ochronosis*

■ **Ankylosing Spondylitis (Marie Strümpel)**

Petrifying / Stiffening of the larger joints – from one end to the other small joints are generally spared

■ **Apophysitis**

If of the tubercles which have been stressed occurs in young athletes who overdo their exercise regimes. Commonest on the Tibia – avulsed bone due to over exercise in the young

Arachnodactyly (Marfan's syndrome)

CT disorder where some LBs are elongated –patients are tall and thin

Arthritis

degenerative

Osteoarthritis

Commonest degenerative arthritis – jt surfaces are have ⬇ cartilage and bone is rubbing on bone causing damage If and pain – large weight bearing jts most vulnerable.

inflammatory

Psoriatica

Associated with Psoriasis autoimmune skin disease – inflamed jts become more painful when the skin symptoms – increase a shifting arthritis

Reactive

Post-infection there may be a reaction in the jts which develop a transient arthritis weeks to months later – w/o the presence of In agent but due to the ⬆ If agents in the BS

Rheumatoid

Autoimmune disease affecting and destroying small joints, with an overgrowth of the synovial membrane

Septic

In agents invading the jts cause If reaction – and may destroy the jt by drawing in If agents and BVs

Arthrogryposis multiplex congenital

congenital multiple jt contractures involving all 4 limbs symmetrically – but there is a lot of variation in the presentation of this rare group of diseases –which do not progress –

Aseptic Necrosis AKA Osteonecrosis

necrosis of a bone or jt w/o an infective agent – generally due to a compromised BS

of the Lunate

The BS & position of the Lunate is such that it is sensitive to trauma in the growing hand and may spontaneously lose its BS – there are 4 stages of wrist degeneration. The resulting death of the bone causes reactive resorption of the surrounding bones & the wrist to develop arthritis and collapse.

Avascular necrosis

Bone death resulting from cessation or compromise of the BS

Baker's cyst see cyst

The herniation of the joint capsule and synovial membrane into the popliteal fossa see the knee examination

Blount's disease see *Tiba vara*

Tibial inward turning – resulting in bow legs

Bone cyst *see cyst*

Unicameral bone cyst – a single radiolucent cyst of bone

Bone infarct *see avascular necrosis*

Brittle bone disease *see osteogenic imperfecta*

Bunion *see also Hallux valgus*

Abnormal enlargement and lateral deviation of the 1st MTP jt

Bunionette (bursitis of the 5th MT)

Abnormal enlargement and medial deviation of the 5th MTP jt

Bursitis

inflammation of a bursa – inflammatory material filling the bursa

Calcific bursitis

inflammation of a bursa – which then calcifies

Olecranon bursitis

large swellings occur at the elbow – when it is constantly weight-bearing or traumatized

Calcaneal spur

outgrowth of bone from the Calcaneus – which is perceptible with weight bearing – relieving the weightbearing will often cause the resolution by dissolution of the bone

Calcifictendinitis

If of the tendon with calcium deposits – occurs mainly in the Achilles tendon

Calve disease *see Vertebra plana*

Carpal tunnel syndrome

the compression of the Ns & tendons in the carpal tunnel – resulting in LOF & pain in the hand

Cerebral Palsy

brain damage resulting in unequal muscle control – causing limb malformation

Cervical rib

supernummery –extra rib arising from C7 – AKA neck rib

Charcot joints *see neuropathic bone & joint disease*

Charcot–Marie-Tooth disease *see pes cavus*

Chondrocalcinosis *see also Gout*

metabolic disorder where calcium deposits are found in jts leading to their destruction - much like gout with uric acid crystals

Chondrodystrophia Calcificans Congenita

this is a mixed group of bony & cartilaginous embryonic malformations. Specific features are: fine stippled, diffuse, dense calcifications In the regions of the epiphyses at any point of the skeleton. The Dx is made on Xray only.

Chondromalacia

softening and roughening of the cartilage

of the Patellae

Internal – tibial surface of the patella – becomes inflamed and then roughened – leading to pain on knee flexion & extension

Club foot *see Talipes equinovarus*

Congenital dislocation of the hip

Generally the head of the femur is malformed or not present and so does not fit into the acetabulum – rarely the acetabulum is too shallow for the femoral head

Congenital High Scapula

A small Coapula is oot too high on the back and so hows outwards and limits the movements of the UL

Congenital Hypercholesteraemia

High serum levels of cholesterol and LDLs which may appear as lumps AKA tendon xanthoma

Congenital short neck AKA Kippel-Fiel syndrome

Characterized by patients with short neck, low hairline, ⬇ neck movement – due to the fusion of 2 or more cervical vertebrae – generally C2-3

Connective tissue disorders

Collection of diseases where collagen is poorly formed or laid down –resulting in fragile bones – misshapen bones and pathological fractures. The disease types range from: hyperelasticity of the skin – cutis hyperelasticus – to osteogenic imperfecta

Coxa Plana AKA Perthes Disease AKA Legge Calve Perthese syndrome

Avascular necrosis of the femoral head occurring in childhood – normal at birth

Coxa Vara *see also slipped femoral head*

Angle b/n the neck of the femur and the hip is ⬇– all diseases encompassing this may be congenital or develop later in childhood

Cyst

Baker's = popliteal herniation of synovium

Bone

aneurysmal

solitary = unicameral bone cyst

Dermoid

implantation cyst

Implantation of skin from a penetration injury which persists and presents as a cyst or swelling – generally in the palm

Synovial = Baker's cyst

De Quervain's tenosynovitis *see tenosynovitis (wrist)*

Dermoid cyst *see cyst*

Diaphyseal aclasis = multiple chondroexostoses

Multiple often connected chondromas – cartilaginous outgrowths from LBs

Discitis

Inflammation of the vertebral discs – swelling and pain with N impingement often result – can occur in any disc as in the disc of the TMJ jt

Dupuytren's disease

Contraction of the flexor tendons in the hand – leading to fixed finger flexion – causes include overuse but may occur spontaneously, associated with carpal tunnel syndrome

Dwarfism *see achondroplasia*

Dyschondroplasia

Enchondromatosis also a general term for malformed cartilage disorders

Dysplasia Epiphysialis Multiplex

Disorder of – 2° growth centres - do not mature normally –presents often as a mild dwarfism

Elher's-Danlos disease AKA Cutis hyperelastica
see Connective tissue disorder

Eosinophilic Granuloma
see Langerhan's cell histiocytosis

Epicondylitis

If of the epicondyles – lat. epicondylitis of the Humerus = tennis elbow / med. = golfer's elbow

Fairbank's disease
see Dysplasia Epiphysialis Multiplex

Femoral anteversion

A developmental rotation of the femoral head – due to uterine position and predisposition >400 may need to corrected, generally fixes itself

Fibromatosis *see neoplasia benign*

Fibrous cortical defect AKA non-ossifying fibroma

Benign well-circumscribed eccentric solitary lesion in metaphysis of LB.

Fibrous Dysplasia

The replacement of normal bone & BM by fibrous tissue & irregular minute bone spicules

Flat foot *see pes planus*

Flurosis

Over-exposure to the Fluride ion causing discolouration in teeth (& bones?) leading to hard brittle bones

Fragilitas ossium *see Osteogenesis imperfecta*

Freiberg's infraction
see osteochondritis of the metatarsals

Frozen Shoulder AKA Adhesive Capsulitis

Giantism *see hyperpituitarism*

Giant cell tumor *see neoplasia – osteoclastoma*

Giant cell tumour of the tendon sheath
see neoplasia synovovioma

Gout

hyperuricaemia leading to deposits in the jts of crystalline deposits

Hallux Rigidus (OA of the big toe)

Hallux Valgus (big toe deviation to the 2nd toe)

Hand-Schuller-Christian disease

see Langerhans histiocytosis

Heberdan's nodes *see Osteoarthritis*

Heel bump / Heel spur *see Calcaneal spur*

Histiocytosis

abnormal proliferation of histiocytes – dendritic & macrophages derived from the BM – when starting from the BM – is called **Langerhans cell hisiocytosis**

Hyperostosis Frontalis Interna AKA Metabolic

Craniopathy

An asymptomatic common, benign thickening of the inner side of Frontalis in women after menopause.

Hyperparathyroidism (Osteitis Fibrosa Cystica)

1°

2°

Hyperpituitarism

adult onset – Acromegaly

infantile onset – Giantism

Hyperthyroidism *see also Osteoporosis*

Hyperviaminosis – excess vitamin doses

A

High doses of vitamin A lead to irregular deposits of cortical bone – particularly the Ulna as well as thin cortical bone & pathological fractures.

D

High doses of Vitamin D even sub-toxic will lead to calcification in Ts and dissecting fibrosis in tendons, which may rupture

Hypophosphatasia

A deficiency of the enzyme alkaline phosphatase – which profoundly affects bone metabolism

Hypopituitarism

varied diseases where 1 of the 8 Hs produced by the gland is deficient most significantly growth H

adult onset

infant onset (Paltuf dwarf)

Infarcts *see avascular necrosis*

Kienbock's disease
see avascular necrosis (of the Lunate)

Kippel-Feil syndrome *see Congenital short neck*

Kohler's disease *see osteochondritis of the Navicular*

Kyphosis

Adolescent kyphosis

Legg-Perthe's disease *see Perthe's disease*

Langerhan's cell histiocytosis

is characterized by radiolucent skeletal lesions of expanded BM areas, which may occur in any bone but generally the skull – it has varying degrees of severity – from single to multiple lesions appearing every 1-2 yrs – and leading pathological #s

Letterer-Siwe disease
see Langerhans cell histiocytosis

Locking finger *see tenosynovitis*

Macrodactyly *see congenital abnormalities*

Marfan's syndrome *see Arachnodactyly*

Metaphyseal Dysostosis

Developmental abnormalities in the metaphyses which often result in short stature

Metatarsus adductus

Inward turning of the foot – resulting in other postural abnormalities

Multiple epiphyseal dysplasia

Diseases of the EP in the bones resulting in abnormal bone growth

Multiple exostoses *see Diaphyseal aclasis*

Muscular dystrophies

Collection of diseases with abnormal muscle development &/or innervation resulting in abonormal postures and bone development

Morquio's syndrome *see Mucopolysaccharidoses*

Morton's neuroma *see Plantar interdigital neuroma*

Mucopolysaccharidoses

Syndrome where long sugars cannot be fully metabolized resulting in abnormal development of bones; kyphosis, bell-shaped chest, coarse facial features, hypermobile jts, knock-knees, large head, short trunk, widely spaced teeth & other abnormalities

Myositis Ossificans

Reactive calcification of the muscles may be mistaken for osteosclerosis

Neoplasia

see bone grid in the main text for full listing

benign

These swellings – Tms are unregulated growth that continue to grow but do not metastasize or invade local Ts – often they have to be removed due to the deformity, pain & LOF they cause. They can be derived from 1 or more of the CTs which make up bone T.

metastatic

The commonest tumours seen in bone are those which originate in other Ts particularly breast, lung & prostate. They are at least 50X greater than 1° bone tumours of any type and occur in older patients.

Neurofibromatosis = *von Recklinghausen's disease*

genetic disorder of the neural crest cells which causes the compact bone to thin, expand and fracture

Neuropathic bone & joint disease

Bones & jts which are insensitive to pain. This results in damage & fractures which go undetected partic important in young immature bones. Some of the primary events causing this are listed below

Charcot jts

Diabetes Mellitus (type II)

Syringomyelia

Tabes Dorsalis

due to sensory N deterioration from Syphilis

Ochronosis

Yellow to black deposits – Alkapton bodies of homogentisic acid due to Alkaptonuria

Olecranon bursitis *see Bursitis*

Ollier's disease *see Dyschondroplasia*

Osteitis fibrosa cystic *see Avascular Necrosis*

Osgood-Schlatter disease see Tibial apophysitis

Osteoarthritis *see also arthritis degenerative*

Osteochondritis Dissecans

Secondary to bone death from lack of BS the articular cartilage is exposed and starved – it flakes off and moves into the jt space leading to arthritis and jt destruction

of the Femur – medial condyle

of the Metatarsals – Freiberg's infarction

of the Navicular

Osteochondrosis – Spinal AKA Scheuermann's disease

Focal disturbance of enchondral ossification in the VC of adolescence slowly crushing the SC and N outlets – i.e. the bone may be poor in original formation or degenerate to cartilage – seen in the VC of adolescents

Osteogenesis Imperfecta = Brittle bone disease

Osteomalacia

adult onset - Paget's disease = Osteitis Deformans

infant onset – Rickets

Osteomyelitis

Osteonecrosis *see Avascular Necrosis*

Osteopetrosis

Osteopoikilosis

Benign, autosomal dominant sclerosing dysplasia of bone characterized by the presence of numerous bone islands in the skeleton, which has numerous white plaques seen throughout the skeleton of equal size.

Osteoporosis (smooth bone atrophy)

Osteosclerosis

Increased bone density either general or localized due to compressing conditions

Paget's disease

Parosteal fasciitis

fibroblastic proliferation with immature woven bone around the periosteum

Peroneal muscular dystrophy *see pes cavus*

Perthe's disease *see Coxa plana*

Pes Cavus

high arch on the foot due to shortened tendons

Pes Planus AKA Flat foot

low or minimal arch on the foot – causing foot pain and compression of the Ns & tendons crossing the sole of the foot

Pigmented villonodular synovitis
see neoplasia benign synovioma

Plantar fasciitis

Heel pain due to If of the plantar fascia/aponeurosis & ligaments severest in the morning when first weight-bearing - no bone growth

Plantar fibromatosis

Fibrous /collagen nodules in the plantar aponeurosis which are painful on weight-bearing – increase with age and do not resolve spontaneously

Plantar interdigital neuroma

Pain in the ball of the foot or forefoot generally 3rd & 4th toes due to benign growth of neural and fibrous T & compression of the Ns in this region

Plantar Spur *see Calcaneal spur*

Pseudo-gout *see Chondrocalcinosis*

Reiter's syndrome *see Arthritis*

Reactive Arthritis *see Arthritis*

Renal osteodystrophy (2º hyperparathyroidism)

Repetitive strain injury *see tenosynovitis*

Rheumatoid nodules *see Arthritis*

Ricket's = hypovitaminosis D *see Osteomalacia*

Sarcoidosis of bone

An inflammatory disorder similar in appearance to TB – but without the In agent. Multiple non-caseating granulomas are found in the LBs & jts causing effusions pain & weakening bones.

Scheuermann's disease AKA adolescent kyphosis

Scoliosis

lateral deviation of the VC

Skeletal Dysplasia

general term for skeletal abnormalities which are present at or soon after birth –Some of these malformations include

absent bones

Achrondoplasia

Ehlers-Danlos syndrome
Fibrous dysplasia

Marfan's syndrome *see arachnodactyly*

Supernumery digits

von Recklinghausen disease
see Neurofibromatosis

Scheuermann's disease *see Osteochondrosis*

Scoliosis = lateral curvature of the spine

Slipped disc = Prolapsed Interevetebral Disc

Slipped femoral head *see Coxa Vara*

One of the many forms of Coxa Vara – due to the avascular necrosis of the head of the femur during development and so dislocating and altering the angle of the hip jt -

Solitary bone cyst *see unicameral bone cyst*

Spina bifida

Failure of the closure of the posterior segments of the VBs

Spondylolisthesis

Anterior or posterior displacement of the VBs on each other – generally in the lumbosaccral region due to bilateral spondylolysis.

Spondylolysis

Malformation or deterioration of the pars articularis of the vertebrae. A term used to describe back pain which it is often associated with, but it may be painless.

Spondylosis deformans

A form of heterotropc bone formation around the VB – osteophytes form around the degenerating VBs

Sprengel's shoulder *see congenital high scapula*

Syndactyly *see congenital anomalies*

Synovitis / Tenosynovitis / Tendonitis

Tarsal tunnel syndrome

The compression of the Ns & tendons in the tarsal tunnel – resulting in LOF & pain in the foot

Tennis elbow *see epicondylitis*

Tenosynovitis

If of the tendons and synovial capsule leading to fixed jts and limited movement

of the 1st dorsal compartment of the wrist

of the finger – trigger finger =
stenosing tenosynovitis = locking finger

Tibia vara AKA Blount's disease

Tibial inward turning – resulting in bow legs

Tibial apophysitis *see Apophysitis*

The avulsion of the immature tibial tuberosity (which has not fully ossified)

Tortcollis = tilting & rotation of the Head

Mainly a meuromuscular disorder where the muscle spasms and deforms the neck – if unchecked bone malformations may develop

Trigger finger *see tenosynovitis*

Unicameral bone cyst *see solitary bone cyst*

Vertebra plana = Calve disease = collapse of VB

Vitamin C deficiency *see Osteoporosis, Scurvy*

Vitamin D deficiency *see Osteomalacia, Rickets*

Von Recklinghausen disease *see Neurofibromatosis*